Healing Codes
Arcturian Sacred Geometry

Nora Hughes

Original Title: Healing Codes – Arcturian Sacred Geometry

This book is a work of non-fiction that explores practices and concepts in the field of spirituality and sacred geometry. Through an intuitive and symbolic approach, the author presents light codes, Arcturian symbols, and spiritual technologies for healing and expanding consciousness.

1st Edition
Production Team
Author: Nora Hughes
Editor: Virginia Santos
Cover: Studios VS / Aruna Delmar
Consultant: Cael Orion
Researchers: Solen Maret, Niah Yuren, Kira Tolmen
Layout: Ilyas Varn

Publication and Identification
Healing Codes – Arcturian Sacred Geometry
VS Publishing, 2025
Categories: Spirituality / Sacred Geometry

DDC: 299.93 – CDU: 133.9

Summary

Systematic Index

consciousness for expansion and travel between realities.

Chapter 7: Dimensional Portals - Discusses portals as points of energetic convergence linking different levels of reality, accessible through vibrational attunement and heightened states of consciousness.

Chapter 8: Sound and Geometry - Explores the intrinsic relationship between sound as the organizing matrix and geometry as the manifest form, revealing how vibration structures reality.

Chapter 9: Codes of Light - Presents light codes as intelligent vibrational patterns transmitted in symbolic form, acting directly on the subtle field for healing, activation, and reconnection.

Chapter 10: Arcturian Healing - Describes the Arcturian approach to healing as a vibrational science that restores inner coherence through sacred geometry, light, and sound, acting on the energy fields.

Chapter 11: Flower of Life - Details the Flower of Life as the primordial pattern of creation, a geometric matrix containing the codes of the universe, acting as a tool for alignment and awakening cosmic memory.

Chapter 12: Golden Ratio - Discusses the Golden Ratio (1.618...) as a universal principle of harmony and beauty present in nature and the cosmos, reflecting divine order in the structure of life.

Chapter 13: Platonic Solids - Introduces the five Platonic solids (tetrahedron, cube, octahedron, dodecahedron, icosahedron) as the geometric pillars of existence, each associated with an element and a specific frequency of consciousness.

Chapter 14: Cosmic Toroid - Explains the toroid as the geometric shape of the continuous flow of energy in the universe, present from particles to electromagnetic fields, representing the self-sustaining cycle of life and consciousness.

Chapter 15: Metatron's Cube - Describes Metatron's Cube as a complex geometric structure derived from the Flower of Life, containing the Platonic Solids and acting as a field for alignment, protection, and access to cosmic records.

Chapter 16: Fractals of Infinity - Explores fractals as self-replicating geometric patterns that structure the universe at all scales, revealing the interconnection between the micro and macrocosm and the infinite nature of creation.

Chapter 17: Arcturian Codes of Peace and Healing - Presents specific geometric codes channeled by Arcturians to restore inner balance, promote peace, and catalyze deep healing processes at energetic and soul levels.

Chapter 18: Symbols of Protection - Details Arcturian geometric symbols that function as vibrational force fields, stabilizing and sealing the energy field against dissonant interferences through the coherence of light.

Chapter 19: Symbols of Healing - Discusses specific symbols that act as light circuits to realign vital frequency, dissolve emotional blocks, and restore energetic integrity, connecting the being to their innate capacity for regeneration.

Chapter 20: Symbols of Manifestation - Explains how geometric symbols act as vibrational codes that organize energy around a clear intention, serving as bridges between the subtle field and materialization in physical reality.

Chapter 21: Symbols of Ascension - Introduces multidimensional symbols that function as light maps and activators of soul memory, facilitating vibrational realignment with the divine essence and evolutionary purpose.

Chapter 22: Journey to the Arcturian Temple - Describes the Arcturian Temple as a vibrational sanctuary in subtle planes, accessible by inner attunement, where healing, learning, and activations occur through light and living geometry.

Chapter 23: Activation of the Cosmic DNA - Explores the concept of a multidimensional DNA containing stellar and spiritual records, detailing Arcturian practices to activate these vibrational layers through light, sound, and geometry.

Chapter 24: Chakra Alignment - Discusses chakras as energy centers with specific sacred geometries, whose alignment through visualization and sound restores vital flow and connection to universal consciousness.

Chapter 25: Daily Rituals - Emphasizes the importance of infusing presence and sacred intention into everyday gestures, transforming simple actions into rituals that anchor light and consciousness daily.

Chapter 26: Sacred Spaces - Discusses the creation of energetically harmonized environments through cleansing, intention, sacred geometry, crystals, and other elements, turning physical spaces into portals of light and connection.

Chapter 27: Collective Planetary Healing - Explores the energetic connection between humanity and Earth, detailing collective practices of sending light, using symbols, and pure intentions to assist in the planet's healing and vibrational upliftment.

Chapter 28: Connection with the Higher Self - Discusses the process of aligning consciousness with its purest, wisest essence through inner silence, deep listening, and practices that dissolve the ego's layers.

Chapter 29: Geometry in Nature - Reveals how the patterns of sacred geometry (spirals, fractals, golden ratio) manifest in all natural forms, from shells and flowers to galaxies, as the language of cosmic intelligence.

Chapter 30: Conclusion and Continuity - Reinforces that the knowledge and activations received are seeds for a continuous path of expansion, spiritual sovereignty, and integration of geometric consciousness into daily life.

Prologue

Somewhere inside you, there is an ancient memory that hasn't been lost—it has merely fallen asleep. A subtle recollection that your existence extends beyond matter, beyond earthly structures and rational explanations.

It is this memory that this book wishes to touch. Not with arguments, but with frequency. Not with theories, but with resonance. Because some books inform, others inspire... and then there are those that activate. This belongs to the last category.

What you hold in your hands is not a compendium of spiritual beliefs or speculations. It is a field. A portal encoded in words, symbols, and sacred geometries, carefully interwoven to create a bridge between the visible and the invisible.

From the very first paragraphs, you might notice something stirring—not outside, but within. A vibration approaching the soul like one recognizing an old friend: silent, loving, and profoundly transformative.

The Arcturians, beings of light originating from one of the most evolved systems in the cosmos, are not mythological characters. They are active consciousnesses, emissaries of cosmic harmony, masters of vibrational healing and living geometry. Their presence is discreet yet unmistakable. Their purpose is not to save, but to mirror. They do not interfere—they remind. They do not lead—they awaken. Their mission is to remind humanity that the light so often sought outside already pulses within.

This book is born as a response to the soul's call. A call that many feel, but few know how to name. It is a map back to the divine origin. Each chapter reveals layers, activates memories, reorganizes internal structures. The words arranged here were chosen with precise intention. They are more than text—they are frequencies. They are codes that interact directly with your energy field, with your spiritual DNA, with the stellar spark that still vibrates silently in your chest.

The sacred geometry, so present in this work, is neither ornament nor abstraction. It is living language. It is the signature of the Source imprinted on every cell, star, or galaxy. The Arcturians understand it as an instrument of healing, alignment, and manifestation. And through it, they build conscious ships, temples of light, chambers of spiritual activation, and structures that respond directly to the pure intention of the being.

You don't need to intellectually understand everything that will be said. In fact, you might discover that the mind will be the last to comprehend—and that's okay. Because this book speaks to the heart. To the light body. To the subtle levels of your being that, silently, have always known. It is a reunion. And like any true reunion, it requires no effort, only presence. Reverence. Breath.

It's not about adopting a new belief. Nor is it about following dogmas or seeking miracles. It's about opening yourself to the experience. About letting inner images reveal themselves, letting dreams intensify, letting symbols begin to appear between the lines of reality. It's about listening to what the soul has always whispered, but the world's haste has muffled.

The Arcturians do not arrive with fanfare. They arrive with light. As you journey through these pages, you will be invited to explore hidden aspects of existence: spiritual technologies, the language of light, activations of the Merkabah field, dimensional portals, and esoteric foundations that support the new consciousness emerging on Earth. Each topic is presented with depth, but also with lightness. Because true knowledge does not weigh down—it liberates.

The transformation will not occur at the end of the reading. It begins now, in this instant. The very moment your eyes rest upon these words, the field is already activated. Because this isn't about reading. It's about feeling. About allowing something new—or perhaps very ancient—to manifest.

You are not alone. And you never have been. Every line of this book has been shaped to vibrate with the same frequency as those who walk beside you on the subtle planes. They watch over you, embrace you, await you. The bridge is open. And the crossing begins with a simple decision: remember who you are.

So, take a deep breath. Let go of control. Open yourself to the unknown with the same confidence as a soul who knows it is returning home. This is not just a book. It is a mirror. And looking into it with an open heart, you will see reflected your purest light.

Chapter 1
Arcturian Introduction

In the cosmic vastness where life pulses in countless forms and dimensions, the Arcturian existence manifests as one of the highest expressions of stellar consciousness active in the multiverse. These beings, originating from the Arcturus system, operate not based on hierarchies or impositions, but in pure harmony with the original matrix of creation. Their presence is subtle, yet profoundly transformative, guided by a wisdom that transcends linear time and is anchored in the frequencies of unconditional love, active compassion, and living geometry. They walk between dimensions, sustaining the balance between worlds and offering, to those whose essence already aligns with the subtlest notes of the universe, the possibility of reconnecting with what was always essential but temporarily forgotten.

Contact with the Arcturians does not occur through conventional means of perception, as their communications happen through patterns of light, sound, and form that interact directly with the subtle fields of being. It is a vibrational exchange that speaks to the soul, reverberating beyond words and reaching deep layers of spiritual memory. Their messages, encoded in geometric structures and languages of light, do not seek to convince or convert, but to remind. To remind of a truth that already dwells within every human being: that we are integral parts of a universal intelligence whose harmony is expressed in perfect geometric patterns. From this perspective, the Arcturians appear not as saviors or external guides, but as living mirrors of our purest potential, resonating with what we are in our divine origin.

The energy radiated by the Arcturians acts as a resonance field that awakens the highest within each individual. Their proposal is not based on beliefs or dogmas, but on direct experience with the frequency of truth. They offer keys to access expanded states of perception, using living symbols and sacred structures that reorganize the observer's vibrational field. By interacting with these forms, consciousness expands naturally, remembering its connection to cosmic cycles, universal archetypes, and the greater purpose of existence. The proposed journey requires not intellectual effort, but sensitive surrender, an open heart, and silent listening. The path is not outside, but within—and the Arcturians are here, like ancestors from tomorrow, to remind us that the light we seek already pulses within us, waiting only for the right moment to reveal itself.

For them, sacred geometry is more than art, more than science—it is the very language of existence. Every line, every curve, every shape holds a spiritual truth. Codes of light that vibrate in resonance with the fundamental patterns of the universe. The flower of life, Metatron's cube, the tetrahedron—these are not mere drawings: they are maps of the invisible, reflections of the divine molded in symmetry. Sacred geometry, from the Arcturian perspective, is not just symbolic; it is operational. It acts, transforms, heals. Each form contains energetic instructions that awaken dormant parts of the being. The spiral activates stellar memories, the circle evokes unity and completeness, the triangle channels energy in a focused way. For the Arcturians, the universe is a symphony of light and form, where everything vibrates in harmony, and where chaos is merely an illusion—a dance not yet understood.

In its origin, human consciousness recognized this language. The ancient Egyptians, the peoples of Atlantis, the Mayan priests, and Andean shamans; all knew that specific forms opened portals, healed ailments, and connected with the gods. The Arcturians silently participated in these civilizations, as mentors and inspirers, radiating their wisdom in dreams, in temples, in the eyes of those who dared to see beyond the veil.

The purpose of this book is to reconnect the reader with this original language. Not as something to be learned mentally, but as something to be remembered spiritually. It offers no doctrines, demands no beliefs. It is a path for those who already feel the call vibrating in their chest, even if they cannot name it. Each chapter will be a key, each symbol a door. By passing through them, one does not find the other—one finds oneself, in one's most expanded, luminous, and real version.

Before proceeding, it is essential to tune into the Arcturian frequency. It is a frequency of purity, inner silence, and unconditional love. For this, we offer a brief opening meditation, a moment of pause where the heart can hear what the ears cannot capture, and the soul can speak without the barriers of the mind.

Sit comfortably, with your spine straight, feet touching the ground. Close your eyes and bring your attention to the center of your chest. Breathe slowly and deeply three times, as if each inhalation brings light, and each exhalation carries away the weight of matter. Now, visualize a bright blue star above your head. It pulses with a soft but intense light, like a distant yet familiar stellar sun. This star is Arcturus. It sends beams of light that descend in golden spirals, touching the top of your head and traveling down your spine. This light cleanses, aligns, awakens.

As you feel this energy, say inwardly: "I open my field to the wisdom of light. I receive the Arcturian frequency with love. May my heart guide this journey." Remain for a few minutes in this state of silent reception. Feel the peace expanding. Feel yourself enveloped by a gentle, loving, timeless presence. The Arcturians need not speak—their vibration already communicates everything. When you feel the time is right, slowly open your eyes. Something has changed. Even if subtly, a new field has been activated around you. A field where the language of light will begin to sketch itself in visions, dreams, sudden inspirations, and synchronicities.

This book is not just a literary work. It is an energy field. Each word has been vibrationally aligned to be more than reading: to be activation. The symbols that will appear along the way are not merely graphics—

they are transmitters, portals compacted into visible forms. They speak to your DNA, to your interdimensional memories, to that part of you that never forgot its origin.

The Arcturians operate with spiritual technologies that do not depend on wires or metals. Their science is made of light and intention. They heal with forms, awaken with tones, elevate with frequencies. When a symbol is contemplated with an open heart, it emits codes. When a geometry is drawn with presence, it becomes a vortex. When an intention is anchored in form, it manifests with divine precision.

The proposed journey requires nothing beyond presence. It doesn't matter if you believe, understand, or know the terms. Vibration precedes comprehension. The soul recognizes what the ego still hesitates to accept. Therefore, trust. If you have come this far, it is because something within you has already begun to align with this call. The Arcturians do not call everyone—only those who, even without knowing, have already answered.

Along the paths to be trodden in the following pages, you will learn to feel, see, hear, and create with the structures of light. Not as an intellectual exercise, but as a return to what is natural, essential, and true. Sacred geometry will reveal its secrets not through logic, but through expanded intuition, subtle perception, the silence that speaks. Each geometric form discussed will be a mirror of the cosmos and a mirror of yourself. Each practice, a remembrance. Each symbol, a note in the cosmic melody that the Arcturians have sung since the beginning of time. And so, step by step, you will realize that ascension is not an escape from Earth, but a full integration with the whole—where spirit and matter, sound and silence, light and shadow intertwine in sacred harmony.

What begins now is more than learning: it is a reunion. The reunion with the primordial language. The reunion with the stellar masters. The reunion with the divine spark that vibrates within you. The language of light has already begun to speak. It draws itself in the space around you, vibrates in invisible patterns, and sings in the geometries of the heart. Everything is ready. And you, now, are too.

Chapter 2
Esoteric Foundations

Long before matter took shape or the word molded the world through language, a silent intelligence was already operating behind the scenes of creation, structuring existence with subtle precision. This intelligence manifests in geometric patterns that not only organize the cosmos but also encode the spiritual principles sustaining life at all levels. Sacred geometry does not arise as a mystical invention or idealization; it is the invisible foundation of reality, the matrix upon which every atom, cell, and star finds its place and purpose. Its origin transcends human time, present since the first whispers of cosmic consciousness, when vibration gave form to light, and light, in turn, became living language. Thus, geometry is not just a visual expression—it is a frequency, a wisdom emanating directly from the creative Source, vibrating in tune with all dimensions of being.

The esoteric understanding of this language goes beyond aesthetics or mathematics. It requires a deep listening to the universe and an inner attunement that recognizes the sacredness of form. Each geometric structure carries an energetic signature, a key capable of accessing expanded states of perception and reconnecting the being to its divine origin. The circle, the triangle, and the spiral are not just recurring figures—they are living archetypes that translate cosmic movements, universal principles, and stages of the spiritual journey. They exist not only in the external world but also reverberate within the human body, reflected in the body's proportions, biological rhythms, mental cycles, and the energy fields surrounding the being. By contemplating these forms with presence and intention, the seeker activates dormant codes in their DNA and awakens ancestral memories of connection with higher planes.

Understanding these foundations is, therefore, much more than an intellectual exercise. It is a process of reconnecting with one's own essence. Geometric forms, when integrated with awareness, become instruments of healing, expansion, and manifestation. They restore the lost alignment between the human and the divine, between the visible and the invisible, between the microcosm and the macrocosm. For the Arcturians, these principles are part of a precise spiritual science, where every line has a function, every angle vibrates with an intention, and every figure is a vortex of universal information. They do not just study geometry—they live within it, like navigators of a reality structured by harmony. By treading this path, the human being rediscovers that they too are a geometric temple in motion, a living mandala dancing with the stars.

These forms are not human inventions. They are revelations. Truths inscribed in the fabric of reality.

Sacred geometry is the calligraphy of the universe. It is how the Source signs its work. When the Arcturians observe the worlds, they do not see chaos or randomness—they see vibrational patterns in perfect harmony, fractal codes repeating on infinite scales, guiding energy towards manifestation. Therefore, understanding geometric foundations is more than studying symbols: it is learning to read the structure of creation.

The circle is the starting point. It represents totality, the unity that precedes duality. It has no beginning or end, and its perfection embodies the essence of the divine. Where there is a circle, there is eternity. The ancients used it to evoke the sacred, to delimit the space between the profane world and the spiritual world. When a circle is drawn, a parallel reality is evoked, a vortex is formed, and linear time gives way to spiral time. This is why spiritual rituals and ceremonies often take place within circles. The Arcturians use this principle to create healing chambers, dimensional portals, and fields of energetic protection. By entering this circular space, consciousness is realigned, as the created vibrational field restores the being's original memory. The circle is the cosmic womb, where the soul can be reborn free from the distortions of density.

The triangle follows, with its power of trinity. It is the first stable structure. It represents spirit, matter, and the consciousness that unites them. Its three points evoke the integration of planes: physical, mental, and spiritual. In the triangle, energy finds direction. The polarity of two finds balance in three. It is the form of ascension, pointing upwards, leading the being from the base to its elevated essence. Ancient temples were built under the influence of this shape. Pyramids, obelisks, and towers follow the triangular principle, not just for aesthetics, but for energetic function. The triangle channels telluric and cosmic energy, linking heaven and earth in a continuous flow. The Arcturians operate with triangles of light to calibrate electromagnetic fields, encode spiritual information, and maintain stability in interstellar ships made not of metal, but of condensed light.

The spiral, in turn, reveals movement. If the circle is being and the triangle is direction, the spiral is the path. Everything in the universe moves in spirals: DNA, hurricanes, solar systems. The spiral is the symbol of evolution, of the eternal return on a higher level. When one walks a spiral, one walks inwards and outwards simultaneously, in a movement that unites introspection and expansion. The spiral does not follow Cartesian logic; it follows the rhythm of the soul. The Arcturians use spirals of energy to deprogram limiting patterns and activate cosmic memories. Each turn of the spiral resonates with a frequency that communicates to the cell its divine origin. It is used for deep healing, as it touches the energetic core of the being, dissolving blockages that even the conscious mind cannot reach.

These three foundations—circle, triangle, and spiral—are the pillars upon which sacred geometry stands. But they are not just figures. They are living, conscious, operative entities. When contemplated with reverence, they awaken dormant perception. When drawn with intention, they create realities. When invoked with voice and presence, they shape the vibrational field around the practitioner.

For the Arcturians, each form is a bridge between worlds. The visible and the invisible touch in the sacred lines of geometry. This is why spiritually advanced civilizations have always used these forms in their architecture, art, and ritual practices. It is no coincidence that megalithic monuments are aligned with constellations. They are mirrors of the heavens on earth, transmitters of stellar codes.

The inner temple is also shaped by these forms. The human body, when analyzed with initiated eyes, reveals itself as a living geometric field. The proportion between bones, heart rhythms, meridian flows—everything follows a pattern. External forms are reflections of internal forms. And by studying sacred geometry, the seeker not only understands the universe but begins to remember who they truly are.

On the spiritual plane, these principles act as keys. Each form possesses a unique energetic signature. By working with these forms, the spiritual being attunes to higher levels of consciousness. It is like tuning a musical instrument: the more precise the form, the purer the vibration. The Arcturians teach that when the human being learns to align their internal structures with sacred forms, they become a channel of pure light. A geometric being, resonant with cosmic harmony.

These knowledges, for eras, were preserved in hidden circles, mystery schools, and initiatic traditions.

The Arcturians, as cosmic guardians of this wisdom, kept the seeds of truth alive, even when humanity strayed from its origin. Today, these seeds germinate again. The time of forgetting gives way to the time of remembrance.

Nothing in this world is random. The flower that opens, the branch that bends, the river that meanders—everything follows a pattern. Apparent chaos is just a part of the design yet unrevealed. Sacred geometry is the lens that allows one to see this design. Not as something separate, but as part of the being. Because the being is geometry. The spirit is form. And consciousness, light organizing itself into patterns.

The foundation has been laid. The fundamentals have been touched. And just as in ancient ceremonies where the ground was traced before the temple was erected, here too the vibrational terrain has been prepared. The circle already pulses around, the triangle points the way, and the spiral spins at the center, connecting the visible to the invisible, the now to the eternal, the reader to the Source.

Chapter 3
Technology of Light

The multidimensional reality surrounding the Arcturians is sustained by an advanced mastery over the principles of light as an intelligent, creative, and transformative force. At their level of consciousness, light is understood as the primary substance of all things, the essential fabric of the universe in its purest form. This understanding surpasses the limits of earthly science and delves into the mysteries of energy as a conscious expression of Creation itself. For the Arcturians, there is no separation between science and spirituality, as both fields are manifestations of the same universal principle: light as the vehicle of divine consciousness.

Their technology, therefore, is not born from the manipulation of inert matter, but from the intentional harmonization of frequencies that shape reality with mathematical precision and sacred beauty. It is a living science, deeply integrated into the cosmic flow, operating through resonance between mind, form, and energy. The technological action of these stellar people does not depend on mechanical tools or external devices, but on the internal activation of vibrational codes latent in all conscious beings. Light, in this context, is not just electromagnetic radiation, but a means of direct communication with the subtlest levels of being. Each technological manifestation is an extension of the vibrational state of the one accessing it, functioning through the attunement between the individual energy field and the harmonic patterns of the universe. The Arcturians interact with these patterns naturally, creating complex systems that instantly align with pure intention. It is a form of engineering based on sacred geometries, harmonic sounds, and colors that speak directly to the soul, configuring structures that organize themselves not by external imposition, but by vibrational coherence with the purpose that animates them. In this way, the technology of light is not a construction separate from the being; it is the extension of its consciousness in manifest form.

This complete mastery over light as technology enables the Arcturians to perform feats that challenge contemporary human logic, such as the materialization of living environments, conscious ships, and dimensional temples. But these feats are not magical or miraculous—they are direct results of a profound understanding of how reality responds to the informational field of consciousness. Everything operates in perfect harmony with the principles of love, wisdom, and unity. By perceiving light as the original matrix of all that exists, the Arcturians become co-creators with the universe, capable of interacting with it not just as observers, but as conscious agents of transformation. This form of knowledge, now offered to humanity, invites each being to awaken their own creative potential, remembering that true technology is found not outside, but within—in the luminous spark that pulses in the heart of every living being.

Light, from the Arcturian perspective, is more than physical illumination. It is the primordial substance of creation. Everything that exists is condensed light at different levels of vibration. When the frequency is high, light remains in subtle, malleable states, moldable by consciousness. When low, it crystallizes into dense, apparent, tangible matter. But the essence remains the same. The technology of light consists in manipulating these frequencies, not with force, but with wisdom, pure intention, and precise geometry. The Arcturians understand the hidden codes of light as one understands the language of the Creator Himself.

Each color, each frequency, each vibration emits an energetic signature. By combining them with specific geometric structures, they create forms of energetic life, healing fields, bioluminescent ships, and dimensional temples. Their constructions are not erected—they are manifested. They arise as extensions of the collective consciousness that conceives them, condensing light and sound into sacred architecture.

What humans call Arcturian ships are, in fact, organisms of conscious light. They do not run on fuels or mechanical mechanisms, but on sacred geometry, toroidal fields, and the crystallization of intention. Each ship is a living expression of the spirit of its people, an emanation of balance and harmony. Its shape is not arbitrary—it is mathematically sacred, designed to resonate with universal patterns of proportion and flow.

Inside these structures, there are no metallic corridors, but spirals of light, living spaces that respond to thought, expanding or contracting according to the vibrational needs of the beings present. The walls sing. The floors emit healing pulsations. The rooms are floating geometries that reorganize according to the purpose of each mission. There, everything is symbiotic. Technology serves consciousness, not the other way around. There is no separation between the being and the instrument: both co-create the experience.

This knowledge is now offered to humanity because Earth has entered a cycle where density begins to yield to light. The third dimension no longer solely supports the evolutionary demands of the soul. It is necessary to integrate subtler technologies that operate not only on the physical but on the energetic and informational field of the being. The Arcturians come as guides, not saviors. They bring vibrational maps, not formulas. And it is up to humans to rediscover within themselves the capacity to use light as a tool for transformation.

This spiritual technology expresses itself on multiple levels. One of the most accessible is vibrational healing. By combining geometric forms with specific frequencies of light and sound, fields are created that restore harmony to cells, chakras, and DNA. A simple crystalline dodecahedron, for example, when activated with violet light and harmonic sound, can reverse deeply ingrained patterns of emotional imbalance. This is not a miracle, but cosmic science applied to the human plane.

Another expression of this technology is stellar education. The Arcturians teach not with words, but with fields of consciousness. They project living holograms, composed of moving geometries, that transmit information directly to the being's light body. This information is assimilated intuitively, as if they were memories resurfacing rather than new data. This is how stellar masters reactivate the ancestral wisdom present in humanity's spiritual DNA.

In the Arcturian chambers of light, which exist on subtle planes of reality, souls in the process of awakening receive specific activations. Each activation is an energetic realignment, a field reprogramming. This can manifest on the physical plane as sudden insights, lucid dreams, emotional releases, or even spontaneous healings. These chambers use fractal patterns, specific colors, and vibrational intonations to lead the being to elevated states of consciousness. They are not accessed by physical ships, but by vibrational attunement. When the being's field is sufficiently harmonized, the connection happens naturally.

The Arcturians also use crystals as amplifiers of light. But these crystals are not just minerals—they are consciousnesses in solid form. Each crystal, when programmed with precise geometric codes, becomes an emitter of highly specific frequencies. It can be used to create protective fields, store information of ancestral wisdom, or anchor the presence of spiritual guides. The crystal functions as a bridge between the physical world and the higher planes.

This science, which seems too advanced for current human understanding, was once lived by ancient civilizations. Atlantis, Lemuria, civilizations of Vedic India, of pre-dynastic Egypt—all knew these technologies. They worked with crystals, sounds, forms, and light. Their temples were built according to cosmic alignments, their practices were rituals of living geometry. But over the millennia, the knowledge became hidden. Not lost—kept. And the Arcturians remained as silent guardians, awaiting the right moment to reactivate it.

Now, that moment has arrived. Light begins to return to Earth in increasing waves of frequency. Those who hear the call feel something awakening within, even if still nameless. They are the ancient engineers of light, the priests of forgotten geometries, the stellar travelers returning to rebuild the temple—not of stone, but of consciousness.

The technology of light is the key to this new era. It will not be dominated by machines, but by awakened hearts. Its functioning depends not on buttons, but on clear intention. It is not controlled—it is co-created. And as more beings attune to these patterns, Earth itself begins to vibrate in another tone, another rhythm, another state of being.

When one contemplates a sacred mandala, when one chants a sound that vibrates in the center of the chest, when one visualizes a geometry enveloped in light and feels their field being realigned—that is using the technology of light. Even if simply, intuitively, it is in this movement that the bridge forms. The Arcturians do not ask for complex rituals. They ask for purity of intention. Where there is love and willingness to serve the light, the technology activates itself.

The journey continues. The light already pulses stronger. And the technology of the spirit begins to reveal its paths to those who walk with the eyes of the heart.

Chapter 4
Language of Light

Interdimensional communication operates from frequencies that directly touch the core of consciousness, allowing exchange between beings from different spheres of existence without the need for conventional words or symbols. The Arcturians master a form of expression that acts as a direct link between cosmic intelligence and the being's vibrational field, a pure language that resonates with the essence, awakening ancestral memories and realigning internal structures. This language does not address the analytical mind, but the subtle field that understands without translating, that recognizes without needing interpretation. It is a living code that speaks to the spirit through forms, colors, sounds, and lights intertwined in patterns of sacred geometry, revealing itself as a system for transmitting universal consciousness.

The language of light acts as a highly encoded vibrational field, structured by higher intelligences who understand the principles of creation in their most elevated form. Each fragment of this language is a vector of energetic information that can reorganize the being's field, bringing healing, expansion, and alignment with divine purpose. When a symbol of light manifests, it is not just an image to be observed, but a field to be experienced. It contains a specific frequency that interacts with the deepest aspects of the being, reconfiguring limiting patterns and activating latent potentials. Unlike human languages, which fragment and translate reality into parts, the language of light presents knowledge in its vibrational totality, where form and meaning are one inseparable thing.

This language operates like a stellar memory imprinted on the soul, capable of being reactivated by simple exposure to its frequency. The recognition of this language is spontaneous, intuitive, like a recollection emerging from the depths of being. It is not learned through intellectual effort, but through an open heart and energetic sensitivity. The human mind may not comprehend the symbols, sounds, or forms presented, but the light body knows what to do with this information. Each contact with these subtle codes is a reunion with the primordial essence, with ancient records that traverse incarnations, dimensions, and forgotten histories. The Arcturians, by sharing this language with humans, are not teaching something new—they are reminding of what was temporarily veiled. By bringing this form of communication to light, they offer not just a means of expression, but a path of reintegration with the totality of being, where consciousness can expand beyond the boundaries of time, space, and form.

Everything that exists vibrates. And this vibration, when it resonates with universal patterns, becomes sound, light, form. Every word spoken, every thought emitted, every emotion felt—all translate into geometric patterns that organize themselves in subtle fields. The language of light is not composed of letters or phonemes, but of forms that sing, colors that speak, structures that touch the heart of consciousness directly. For the Arcturians, this language is the matrix of reality. It is with it that they build their knowledge, their communications, and their fields of teaching.

Unlike verbal communication, which separates, classifies, and interprets, the language of light unifies. It speaks not to the intellect, but to the essence. When a symbol of light is emitted, it activates dormant frequencies in the recipient's vibrational field. There is no need for explanation—there is only recognition.

This form of communication is not exclusive to the Arcturians. Earth civilizations, in their golden ages, also mastered this language. In ancient Egypt, hieroglyphs were not just writings—they were vibrational portals. Each symbol carried an energy field that interacted with whoever contemplated it. In the Vedic tradition, yantras functioned as energetic maps and tools for deep meditation. Tibetan mandalas, Mayan inscriptions, Nordic runes—all are fragments of this universal language, remnants of a wisdom that was not lost, but fell asleep in humanity's collective unconscious.

Philosophers like Pythagoras and Plato did not just study mathematics and forms—they glimpsed the sacred link between number, sound, and form. Pythagoras claimed that everything is number, but he referred not to number as an abstract concept, but as the ordering vibration of the cosmos. He saw in musical intervals a direct correspondence with geometric proportions. For him, the universe was a harmony—a silent sacred music, where each being plays a note. Plato, in turn, spoke of the world of ideas, where pure forms reside. The Platonic solids, which he studied, are geometric manifestations of these original ideas. Each is a perfect expression of universal symmetry, corresponding to the elements of nature and the dimensions of the soul. Both thinkers, even without modern vocabulary, touched the veils of this primitive language—the same one the Arcturians master fully.

When one comes into contact with a symbol of light, one is not just facing an image. One is facing a transmitter of consciousness. The Arcturians channel these forms as tools for awakening. Each symbol contains a specific frequency aimed at an aspect of the being: emotional healing, chakra alignment, spiritual DNA activation, energetic protection, perception expansion. They are maps for the soul to navigate through the layers of time and dimensions.

These codes are alive. They transform according to the vibrational field of the one accessing them. The same symbol can have different effects on different people, as it interacts with the field uniquely. And even within the same being, it manifests in diverse ways according to the moment, intention, inner state. The language of light is dynamic. It breathes, pulses, evolves with the consciousness that contemplates it.

When working with these codes, the being doesn't need to mentally understand their meanings. The simple act of contemplating, drawing, chanting, or meditating with them is enough for the effects to manifest. The mind might resist, try to decipher, doubt—but the heart will know. The soul recognizes what the mind forgot. And that is why the language of light is so powerful: it bypasses the rational filter and speaks directly to what is true within us.

This language is not limited to visual form. It also expresses itself in sounds, movements, colors, and even sensations. When one chants an intuitive mantra, when the body moves in spontaneous dances, when the light of a crystal touches the skin and evokes an inexplicable emotion—in these moments, the language of light is at work. It is synesthetic. It permeates all layers of experience.

The Arcturians teach that for this language to be reactivated to its full potential, it is necessary to open the higher channels of perception. This means clearing the filters of the mind, healing emotional traumas that block energy flow, and aligning the vibrational field with elevated states of consciousness. It is not an effort of study, but a path of inner transformation.

Practicing with sacred geometry is one of the most effective ways to initiate this reactivation. By contemplating a sacred form with presence and intention, the energy field reorganizes. Ancient dormant codes begin to emit light. The spiritual DNA, containing records of other lives, dimensions, and stellar lineages, starts to open like a book of forgotten wisdom. The language of light, then, begins to emerge not as something new, but as something that was always there, waiting to be remembered.

Some awakened beings have already begun channeling this language in new forms. Paintings with unknown symbols, automatic writings that follow no earthly alphabet, intuitive songs in languages belonging to no nation. These are signs of the return of the original language. It will not come with grammars or translations, but with vibration and recognition. And the more it is used, the clearer it will become.

It is possible to start integrating this language into daily life. Visualizing geometric forms during meditation, intuiting sounds that spontaneously arise in the throat, letting the hands freely draw symbols that appear in visions—all are ways to bring the language of light to the surface. It is not necessary to understand—it is necessary to feel. Trust what resonates, follow what vibrates, allow the soul to guide the process.

The Arcturians stand beside those who open themselves to this reconnection. They do not impose, do not instruct linearly. They radiate. They envelop the seeker's field with specific frequencies. And when the seeker is ready, the codes begin to be received. Vivid dreams, synchronicities, symbols appearing repeatedly in daily life—all are subtle forms of the language of light initiating dialogue with the awakened consciousness.

This language is the link between worlds. It allows access to higher planes of existence, reception of teachings directly from the source, holographic understanding of reality. It is the bridge between the human and the divine, between what is seen and what is felt, between what one is and what one can be. By allowing the language of light to reveal itself, a path of return opens. Return to origin, to remembrance, to the greater purpose. Words fall silent. Forms speak. And the being, now expanded, begins to listen to the invisible symphony of the cosmos that has always been singing its name.

Chapter 5
Energetic Preparation

Spiritual ascension occurs with stability only when there is consistent energetic preparation, rooted in conscious and committed practices. Interaction with elevated frequencies, such as those manifesting through sacred geometry, the language of light, and Arcturian codes, requires an energy field previously structured to accommodate such manifestations. The subtle energy permeating these codes acts directly on the most delicate bodies of the human being—the subtle bodies—which, by their very nature, are sensitive to the vibrational influences of the environment, thoughts, and emotions. When this internal system is misaligned, overloaded, or fragmented, it not only hinders the absorption of higher frequencies but also creates resistance to the transformative processes these energies promote. Thus, more than desiring or visualizing connection with higher planes, it is imperative to create the internal conditions that enable this interaction in a fluid, stable, and integrated manner.

The Arcturians deeply understand the vibrational structures and mechanisms regulating the relationship between dimensions. According to their guidance, energetic preparation is not a luxury but a basic requirement for spiritual activation processes to occur harmoniously. They emphasize that spiritual energy, upon contacting the human field, amplifies everything it encounters: both light and shadow. Therefore, if the field is polluted, unstable, or weakened, internal distortions are intensified and can compromise the evolutionary process. Conversely, when the energy system is clean, anchored, and protected, light penetrates clearly, acts deeply, and facilitates the integration of new information, frequencies, and consciousnesses. Energetic preparation, then, is not just a protective resource but a form of respect for one's own spiritual journey, an act of self-love and love for the greater purpose one wishes to manifest.

This preparation involves recognizing energetic reality as being as concrete as material reality. It means understanding that spiritual life does not happen apart from daily life but within it, permeating every gesture, thought, and feeling. To anchor oneself is to be present in existence with responsibility and openness. To cleanse oneself is to liberate oneself from the burdens that obscure the perception of one's own light. To protect oneself is to delimit the sacred space where the spirit can flourish. And to attune oneself is to vibrate at the frequency of inner truth, the one that resonates with higher planes and sustains communication with benevolent and evolved intelligences. When a being performs this preparation consistently and dedicatedly, spirituality ceases to be a concept and becomes a real experience. The Arcturian codes, once mere geometric forms, become mirrors of the soul itself. And the spiritual journey ceases to be a search and becomes recognition—of something that, in essence, has always been present.

Every human being carries within them a complex energetic mesh, composed of multiple levels of existence: physical, emotional, mental, spiritual. These levels are interconnected by vortices that spin in spirals—the chakras—and sustain the flow of vital energy. When there are traumas, limiting beliefs, dense emotions, or repetitive thoughts, this system becomes unbalanced. Energies do not circulate fluidly. They accumulate, stagnate, cause disconnection. And in the absence of flow, there is no integration of light. Therefore, before diving into the codes of sacred geometry, it is necessary to cleanse, align, and strengthen this field.

The first step is anchoring. Anchoring is establishing a conscious connection with the Earth. It is recognizing the physical body as a temple, the ground as support, incarnate life as purpose. Many spiritual seekers fail because they try to ascend without rooting. They want to reach higher planes without stabilizing their base. The Arcturians teach that the higher the expansion, the deeper the rooting must be. Light cannot sustain itself in the air. It needs body, presence, ground. To anchor, full presence in the now is required. Sit in silence, with bare feet touching the soil. Visualize roots of light emerging from the soles of your feet, penetrating deep layers of the earth, connecting to the planet's crystalline core. Breathe consciously, feeling the gravitational force as an ally, not a prison. The Earth is a living being. And by connecting with it, a network of energetic support is activated that stabilizes the personal field and allows the safe reception of elevated frequencies.

With anchoring established, the next step is cleansing. The subtle bodies accumulate vibrational residues from thoughts, emotions, environments, and interactions. These energies, if not regularly purified, become blockages. Energetic cleansing can be done in various ways, but the Arcturians recommend using violet light as a universal transmuter. Violet light acts like a cosmic fire, burning away densities and converting them into consciousness. Visualize a spiral of violet light descending from above, enveloping your entire body. Feel this spiral spinning, penetrating pores, organs, energy centers. It travels through the channels, dissolves miasmas, releases ancient crystals of pain. Breathe deeply during the process. Each exhalation carries away what no longer serves. And each inhalation brings renewal. At the end, visualize yourself completely immersed in a field of pure, clear, subtle light.

Energetic protection follows. Opening oneself to light also means becoming more sensitive to surrounding fields. Not all energy is compatible. Not all presence is beneficial. The energy field, when exposed without protection, can be invaded by unbalanced frequencies that drain vitality and confuse perception. The Arcturians use specific geometries to create protective shields. Among them, the octahedron stands out—a shape composed of two opposing pyramids, generating a balanced field in all directions. Visualize yourself inside an octahedron of golden light. Feel its vertices connecting to the cardinal points, to the sky, and to the earth. This field repels what does not resonate with your essence. It allows entry only to elevated frequencies. It is an intelligent vibrational filter, tuned to your higher intention. Whenever starting a spiritual practice, reactivate this structure. It will keep you centered, stable, and at peace.

The final stage of preparation is vibrational attunement. It is at this point that the field is elevated so that communication with higher planes occurs clearly and safely. The Arcturians operate at frequencies far beyond the density of the third dimension. To perceive them, one must raise one's own vibration. This can be done through conscious breathing, sacred sound, and light visualization. Start with breathing: inhale slowly, counting to eight, hold for four, exhale counting to eight, and remain without air for another four. Repeat this cycle several times. It regulates the nervous system, harmonizes heartbeats, and synchronizes the electromagnetic field with universal rhythms. Next, chant the sound "OM" or another intuitive sound that arises. Vocal perfection doesn't matter—what matters is the intention. Sound activates the vibrational field. It creates internal resonance. Sound shapes light. And when light and sound align, geometry appears. Now, visualize a point of stellar blue light above your head. This is the point of contact with the Arcturians. From it, a spiraling beam of light descends, touching the top of your head, moving down the spine, activating the chakras, penetrating the heart. Feel this light as a conscious, loving, welcoming presence. It does not impose, does not judge—it simply radiates. Allow yourself to be filled by it.

This attunement need not last long. A few minutes are enough for the field to align. And at the end, remain in silence. Listen to what cannot be heard. Feel what cannot be said. This is the Arcturian frequency. It does not arrive with fanfare. It arrives with serenity.

With the field anchored, cleansed, protected, and attuned, the being is prepared. The geometries that previously seemed like mere drawings now vibrate. The symbols come to life. The practices become portals. Not because something external changed, but because the interior has been calibrated. The channel is open. The Arcturians emphasize that energetic preparation is not a mechanical ritual, but an internal stance. It is the act of revering the sacred. Of remembering that every spiritual practice is an encounter with the Source. And like every encounter with the divine, it requires presence, respect, and openness.

The field is ready. The light awaits. And the being, now aligned, becomes a receptacle for the truth that has always been theirs.

Chapter 6
Active Merkabah

There exists a vibrational field intrinsic to the human being, profoundly connected to the essence of life and the structure of reality, which transcends the limits of matter and common perception. It is a subtle and complex architecture, activated not by technological devices, but by consciousness in a high state of coherence. This field, known as the Merkabah, manifests as an interdimensional vehicle whose origin dates back to stellar civilizations and ancestral spiritual traditions. It is neither a symbolic invention nor a philosophical allegory, but a real energetic structure, present in the light body of every human being, whose function is to facilitate the expansion of consciousness and movement between different levels of reality. The Merkabah operates as a bridge between the physical and the ethereal, between the now and the eternal, activating in response to the individual's vibrational alignment with the harmonic laws of the universe.

The presence of the Merkabah in the human field is encoded in sacred geometry and sustained by universal principles governing the flow of cosmic energy and information. Its activation occurs when there is full integration between mind, heart, and spirit, allowing light to travel through the subtle channels of the energy body with fluidity and intelligence. Unlike any external technology, the Merkabah requires no physical components, but rather internal states of purity, clear intention, and deep connection with the Higher Self. Its functioning is directly related to the practitioner's consciousness and their willingness to live their inner truth authentically. When activated, the Merkabah creates a toroidal field around the body, which not only protects and elevates but also connects the individual to high-vibration frequencies, facilitating communication with higher planes and access to cosmic records of wisdom.

The structure of the Merkabah reveals a principle of union between complementary polarities—masculine and feminine, heaven and earth, spirit and matter. Its two intertwined tetrahedrons spinning in opposite directions form a dynamic vortex of light that pulses in resonance with the matrix of creation. This rotation is not just a visual representation but a real movement of subtle energies that reorganizes the being's vibrational field, harmonizing the physical, emotional, mental, and spiritual bodies. The Merkabah, when fully activated, becomes a self-aware field, a living presence that responds to the practitioner's intention and acts as an extension of their soul in communion with the cosmos. It is a process of remembrance and reunion with one's own divine nature, in which the light body awakens and integrates into the stellar mesh of existence, making the human being a conscious traveler between worlds.

The word Merkabah carries three roots of ancient origin: "Mer," representing light; "Ka," representing spirit; and "Bah," representing body. It is the union of these three forces that constitutes the Merkabah field: an interdimensional vehicle capable of transporting consciousness between realities, connecting subtle planes, and accessing cosmic records that lie beyond the veils of ordinary perception. All great esoteric traditions mention, under different names and symbols, the existence of this ascension vehicle. But it is with the Arcturians that this knowledge is revealed in a practical and experiential way.

The Merkabah is composed of two interpenetrating tetrahedrons that spin in opposite directions, creating a toroidal field around the body. One tetrahedron points upwards, representing masculine, solar, active energy, the ascending spirit. The other points downwards, symbolizing feminine, lunar, receptive energy, matter opening to the divine. When both spin in perfect harmony, a spiral of light is created, and the being is enveloped by a living, conscious structure that resonates with universal intelligence.

In ancient times, this activation happened naturally, as humanity lived in greater alignment with cosmic rhythms. But with the accumulation of mental, emotional, and energetic density, this vehicle became deactivated in the collective field. It remained latent, dormant like a seed beneath the earth. Now, with the return of stellar frequencies to Earth, the Merkabah begins to awaken again in beings who align with the call of light.

The activation of the Merkabah is not an external event. It is an internal process that requires preparation, presence, and vibrational purity. The Arcturians teach that the key to this activation lies in clear intention and the state of coherence between heart and mind. There is no imposition, no force. The Merkabah responds to the internal field, to the being's resonance. When there is harmony, it forms. When there is truth, it spins. And when it spins, it transports the soul beyond the limits of time.

Visualizing the Merkabah is the first step. Sit in silence, breathe deeply, and visualize two tetrahedrons of translucent light in your field. One with its base on the ground and its vertex pointing to the sky; the other with its base facing upwards and its vertex towards the earth. Both intersect at your heart center. Feel these tetrahedrons spinning, each in its own direction, creating a vortex of light around you. The rotation should be harmonious. The upper tetrahedron spins clockwise, and the lower, counterclockwise. There is no need to force the visualization—clear intention is enough. Energy organizes itself according to consciousness. As the practice progresses, you will feel an expansion. The body seems to vibrate, the space around changes, and a subtle yet potent field envelops you completely. This is your Merkabah awakening.

With the Merkabah active, perception changes. Sounds become deeper, colors gain new nuances, insights emerge like forgotten memories returning to the surface. This occurs because the Merkabah acts as a cosmic antenna, capturing information from higher planes and translating it to the practitioner's field. Each rotation is a code. Each rotation is a frequency. Each rotation is a portal.

The Arcturians use the Merkabah not only as a means of interdimensional transport but also as a tool for healing, protection, and expansion. When activated correctly, the Merkabah cleanses energy fields, restructures spiritual DNA, and protects against low-vibration interferences. In situations of vibrational challenge, simply visualizing the Merkabah spinning is enough for a shield to form and the field's integrity to be restored.

There are advanced practices involving sound, breath, and movement to intensify Merkabah activation. Specific vowel tones can be chanted during visualization, especially the sounds "RA," "SA," "KA," which resonate with higher energy centers and facilitate harmonic rotation. Breathing should be rhythmic, deep, connecting heaven and earth with each cycle. Over time, the Merkabah ceases to be a practice and becomes a constant presence—a self-sustaining field of living light.

Some practitioners report profound experiences after activating the Merkabah: lucid dreams with stellar symbols, visions of light temples, sensations of floating outside the body, telepathic communications with beings of high consciousness. These phenomena are not illusions or products of fantasy—they are legitimate manifestations of an expanded field. The Merkabah is the portal through which the soul remembers its stellar origin. It also allows conscious access to the Akashic Records—the cosmic library where all memories, lives, and experiences are stored. By traveling with the Merkabah, the soul can visit planes where pure knowledge resides, without distortions. There, it does not learn—it remembers. And upon returning to the body, it brings back the light of truth that illuminates the path.

Activating the Merkabah does not replace the spiritual path—it intensifies it. It is a catalyst. It reveals what needs transformation, amplifies what is hidden, accelerates what is gestating. That is why, for many, the awakening of the Merkabah is accompanied by processes of emotional purification, memory healing, and purpose realignment. The light it radiates allows no self-deception. It shows everything.

Therefore, the Arcturians advise: do not rush. Respect the inner rhythm. Activate your Merkabah with love, reverence, surrender. Each practice is an initiation. Each spin, a seed planted in consciousness. Over time, the vehicle of light will become as familiar as the body itself. And then, there will no longer be separation between here and beyond, between human and stellar, between what one is and what one has always been. The Merkabah is more than a tool—it is a state of being. When active, the personal field resonates with the harmony of the universe. The being becomes one with the geometry of creation, a conscious point of light navigating the worlds as an emissary of the Source. In this state, there is no fear. There is remembrance. There is expansion. There is living presence in the eternal now.

The journey continues. The light spins. And the sacred vehicle awakens, leading the soul to reunite with its origin of stars.

Chapter 7
Dimensional Portals

The structure of the universe is interwoven with points of energetic convergence that operate beyond ordinary perception, acting as true links between different levels of reality. These points, known as dimensional portals, exist as specific frequencies that interconnect subtle planes and cosmic accesses, and their activation depends on the being's vibrational state. The Arcturians understand these portals not as metaphors, but as tangible realities that respond directly to awakened consciousness. They manifest in places of strong energetic resonance on Earth and also within the internal centers of the human body, reflecting the unity between the macrocosm and the microcosm. The nature of these portals is not physical, but vibrational, revealing that true access is conditioned not by spatial displacement, but by the elevation of the state of being.

The reality of a portal lies not in its appearance, but in its function: to be a bridge between dimensions. Each portal pulses with a unique energetic signature, which can only be decoded through conscious attunement with its frequencies. It is a dance between sacred geometries, clear intentions, and states of full presence. Portals respond to harmony, the coherence of the internal field, and the spiritual maturity of the practitioner. There is no external mechanism that opens them, as their activation is always a reflection of internal readiness. When a being aligns with their essence, purifies their emotions, and silences their thoughts, they become a living key that resonates with the doors of the invisible. The portal, then, not only reveals itself—it invites, recognizes, welcomes.

This interaction between portals and consciousness is not unilateral: upon crossing a portal, the human being not only receives—they also transmit. They carry their frequency, purpose, light to planes that often await precisely this interaction to complete cycles of healing, learning, or expansion. The crossing is always an act of co-creation. Therefore, accessing a portal is not an act of escaping physical reality, but an extension of the spiritual journey, where the explorer becomes an ambassador of consciousness in multiple realities. Earth is filled with these access points, silently active in certain locations and dates, and also in the recesses of the human body and soul. Connecting with these portals requires responsibility, discernment, and reverence, as each passage represents an opportunity for reconnection with the vastness of being.

For the Arcturians, portals are not myths, but living structures of the universe. They exist at specific points on Earth, marked by ancient monuments, natural formations, and cosmic alignments, but also exist within the human being—in the heart, the pineal gland, the upper chakras. They are resonant geometries that, when activated by clear intention and elevated vibrational state, reveal dimensions coexisting with this one, but vibrating at subtler levels of reality.

Each portal responds to a geometric configuration. They are not physical doors hidden in caves or mountains, but patterns activated in specific energetic contexts. Pyramids, for example, are portals. Stone circles, ancient labyrinths, sacred caves, and certain temples built with harmonic proportions are too. But the real key is not the location, but the state of the being. It is the practitioner who transforms into the vibrational password that activates the portal.

Sacred geometry acts as a catalyst in this process. When a geometric pattern is visualized or drawn with presence and intention, it begins to reorganize the surrounding energy field. If this form resonates with a specific dimensional point, it can generate a vortex, a temporary opening where time bends, light condenses, and new perceptions become possible. The Arcturians use specific stellar mandalas to access these points. Each mandala is a map. Each symbol, an interdimensional coordinate.

But for the portal to reveal itself, the field must be prepared. Energetic preparation, alignment with the Merkabah, and activation of the language of light are not isolated rituals—they are steps preceding entry into expanded states of consciousness. When working with portals, the being needs to be stabilized. Otherwise, what should be a crossing can become disorientation. The light passing through the portal amplifies everything it touches. And if there is internal noise, it will be multiplied. Therefore, the Arcturians recommend specific practices before any attempt to contact portals.

The first is inner silence. Not the silence of absence of sounds, but the silence of absence of mental noise. When the mind quiets, intuition manifests. And it is intuition that guides the being through the paths of the invisible. Next, presence. Being whole in the moment, with full attention to the body, breath, the surrounding field. Full consciousness is the greatest instrument of interdimensional navigation.

Guided visualizations are powerful tools for accessing portals. They are not mere imaginations—they are directed projections of consciousness that can touch higher realities. A common Arcturian practice consists of visualizing a circular portal before oneself, composed of white and blue light, with symbols vibrating on its edge. By fixing the inner gaze on this portal, the practitioner chants a sound that intuitively arises from the chest, sustaining the vibration. Gradually, a sensation of displacement begins. Space changes, time slows down, and a new energetic landscape presents itself. This landscape might be a temple, a stellar garden, a sphere of light, or simply an immersion in floating geometric patterns. What lies beyond the portal depends on the practitioner's frequency and purpose.

Some souls are led to spiritual councils, where Arcturian masters and other beings of light share guidance in silence, through gazes, gestures, or direct information transfer. Others are taken to healing chambers, where specific vibrational patterns restore energetic balance at all levels of the being. The cosmic records can also be accessed through portals. These are informational fields where all the soul's experiences are archived as encoded light. By crossing a portal designated for this purpose, the practitioner can receive visions of past lives, probable futures, choices made in other parallel realities. These accesses are not for spiritual entertainment, but for integration. They offer pieces of the puzzle of spiritual identity, helping the being remember who they are and why they are here.

There are portals that open only at specific cosmic moments. Planetary alignments, eclipses, solstices, and equinoxes activate specific geometries on Earth and in the subtle bodies. The Arcturians, attentive to these cycles, guide seekers to practice specific meditations during these periods. On these occasions, the veils between worlds become thinner, and the crossing becomes more fluid. These moments should not be wasted, as they contain the potential for quantum leaps in consciousness.

Portals are not just entryways—they are also emission pathways. The being accessing these realities also emits vibration into them. When someone crosses a portal with a pure heart and intention of service, their presence brings light to the planes they visit. Therefore, the crossing is never unilateral. It is always an exchange, a co-creation between dimensions. The Arcturians teach that each visit to a portal is also a seeding. And that every seed of light planted in another dimension returns to Earth as the fruit of wisdom.

It is important to understand that portals need not be sought in distant places. The point between the eyebrows, the center of the heart, the base of the spine—all are internal portals. They connect to the Higher Self, to stellar lineages, to spiritual mentors. By concentrating attention on these points during meditation, the practitioner can feel the opening of a field, the expansion of perception, the reception of subtle instructions. The journey is not outward—it is inward. And by diving within oneself, the being touches the infinite.

Some portals remain open for long periods; others close soon after access. There are permanent portals and temporary portals. There are natural portals and intentionally constructed portals. There are those that lead to planes of light and those that lead to intermediate zones of purification. Therefore, discernment is essential. The portal's frequency can be felt. If there is fear, heaviness, confusion, one should not cross. But if there is peace, clarity, lightness, it is a sign that the crossing is safe.

Over time, with constant practice, the practitioner begins to feel portals in their daily presence. A place in the house becomes sacred. A tree on the path reveals itself as a guardian. A mirror becomes a symbol of passage. Reality becomes holographic, and the visible world begins to reveal its hidden layers. The being transforms into a conscious dimensional traveler, carrying within them the living map of the paths of light.

The Arcturians observe with joy when a human being consciously crosses a portal. For them, it is a sign of spiritual maturity, of returning to the cosmic home. They do not intervene, do not pull—they simply radiate the frequency. The portal forms when the being is ready. And each step taken in light is celebrated on the subtle planes with reverent silence and unconditional love.

Dimensional portals are not fiction. They are subtle reality, available to those who dare to see beyond form. They are here, now, vibrating silently around, waiting for the being to remember the password: presence, purity, purpose. Light is the door. The heart, the key. And the traveler, the one who awakens to the infinite within themselves.

Chapter 8
Sound and Geometry

At the core of reality, sound manifests as the organizing matrix that structures all existing forms. It is not just a wave propagating through air, but a creative power acting silently, shaping the invisible substance of the universe with precision and purpose. In its purest essence, sound operates as the primordial architect of matter, gathering dispersed particles into coherent patterns that manifest as visible and tangible geometries. It is through vibration that energy condenses into form, revealing the intimate relationship between the inaudible and the visible. This continuous interaction between frequency and structure shows that creation is not a static act, but a dynamic process of resonance, where each emitted sound reorganizes light into harmonious configurations that mirror the consciousness that generated it.

Sound, in this context, transcends its physical aspect and reveals itself as a universal language, capable of communicating directly with the subtle fields of existence. It acts simultaneously on the emotional, mental, spiritual, and physical planes, being felt as pulsation, visualized as color and form, and intuitively understood as truth. In advanced cultures like the

Arcturians', sound is an agent of conscious transformation, used to sculpt reality and align the being's frequencies with the original cosmic patterns. The emission of specific tones, calculated with mathematical precision, allows energy to be directed with intention and clarity, generating vibrational fields that activate geometric structures on the subtle plane. These forms do not just represent ideas or symbols; they are living organisms, pulsars of consciousness that organize the surrounding energetic space into mandalas of balance and expansion.

The relationship between sound and geometry, therefore, is not merely conceptual, but experiential. When a pure sound is intoned with presence and purpose, it reorganizes the surrounding field into precise figures reflecting natural laws of proportion, harmony, and symmetry. This ability of sound to generate form is at the base of ancestral practices that understood the universe as a symphony in motion, where each vibrational expression is connected to an invisible architecture of energy. By accessing this principle, the human being reconnects with ancient and profound knowledge, in which every emitted note, every sustained frequency, is an invitation to reconnect with the divine matrix of creation. In this space of conscious listening and true expression, sound and geometry dance together, revealing the sacred code that sustains all things.

When creation began, there was no word—there was vibration. The initial vibration, dense with intention and consciousness, reverberated through layers of realities, generating ripples that became forms. Form, therefore, is condensed sound. What the eyes see as structure, the invisible ear hears as song. The flower, the shell, the snowflake—all are notes of a cosmic score revealing itself in harmonic proportions. When the sound is pure, the resulting form is also pure.

On Earth, ancient civilizations understood this link between sound and geometry. Vedic mantras, Gregorian chants, Egyptian hymns, shamanic drums—all were more than cultural expressions. They were access keys. Each ritualistic sound was emitted with precision, charged with intention and resonance. In temples where acoustics were shaped according to golden proportions, voices generated vibrational fields so potent they altered states of consciousness. Sound became form. Form, the vehicle of spirit.

The Arcturians master this principle expertly. They use precise intonations to activate light codes, stabilize energy fields, and transmit interdimensional information. When communicating with humans, they often do so through sounds belonging to no earthly language. They are pure vibrations, modulated with mathematical precision, penetrating the recipient's field like spirals of sonorous light. The effect is not just auditory—it is cellular, energetic, holistic.

Each Arcturian sound is also a living geometry. By emitting a frequency, they simultaneously project a corresponding geometric form. This synesthesia is essential in their communication. Sound and form are not separate—they are different expressions of the same energy. A specific sound might generate a vibrant dodecahedron in the being's field, another might activate a rotating toroid. These forms, in turn, restructure the energy field and release blockages hindering vibrational ascension.

This practice can be integrated into the path of the earthly seeker. Intuitive intonation is one of the most accessible and potent tools for generating geometric forms in the energy field. It's not necessary to know how to sing, nor understand music. The sound that heals is not the tuned one, but the true one. When sound spontaneously springs from the heart, without judgment, it carries the soul's original vibration. And this vibration, upon being emitted, organizes the surrounding light into sacred patterns.

A simple practice consists of silencing the inner space, aligning the breath, and allowing a sound to emerge intuitively. This sound can be prolonged, pulsating, high or low pitched. The important thing is to sustain it with presence. Simultaneously, visualize a geometric form taking shape before you—a circle, a star, a spiral. Feel the resonance between the sound you emit and the form you see. Over time, this practice refines. Sound guides form. Form shapes the field. And the field responds with expansion.

Crystals can also be used as amplifiers in this process. Emitting sounds near specific crystals, like quartz, selenite, or moldavite, makes the generated patterns clearer and more intense. Crystals absorb, modulate, and re-emit sound as coherent geometry. In Arcturian healing sessions, it's common to find crystals arranged in geometric patterns around the practitioner, while specific intonations are emitted by beings of light or reproduced by non-physical vibrational devices.

The human body, in turn, is an instrument of resonance. Each organ, each bone, each cavity is an acoustic chamber. When emitting sounds, the vibration reverberates internally, stimulating energy points and activating subtle geometries. The heart, for example, responds to deep sounds with openness. The pineal gland, to high-pitched sounds. When these sounds are emitted in sync with geometric visualizations, a toroidal field is created connecting the chakras, aligning the meridians, and expanding the light body.

Arcturian vocalizations follow numerical patterns corresponding to the Fibonacci sequence, the golden ratio, and harmonic intervals. A sound repeating in multiples of eight, for instance, tends to generate spiral patterns reminiscent of DNA. Vocalizations based on the 3-6-9 sequence—as intuited by Nikola Tesla—tend to activate multidimensional structures of the field, connecting the being to elevated frequencies of the stellar plane.

But not only vocal sound is effective. Intuitive instruments, like Tibetan bowls, ocean drums, wind chimes, and crystal harps, also act as sonic sculptors. When played with intention, they produce waves that draw invisible geometric shapes in the environment. These shapes remain in the space for a considerable time, influencing the vibrational field even after the sound ceases. The Arcturians teach that every true sound leaves a trail of light. And this trail is a living form.

Singing within a mandala, chanting mantras before a Flower of Life, or vocalizing sacred tones while visualizing Metatron's Cube are practices that create synergy between sound and geometry. In this state, the being becomes the temple itself. Each cell vibrates in harmony with the cosmic structure. And consciousness expands beyond the mind, beyond the body, beyond history.

Sound healing is not just a possibility—it is a necessity in times of planetary transition. The excess of artificial noises, electromagnetic pollution, and the bombardment of disordered information fragment the human field. Sacred sound, conversely, reorganizes. It returns the being to its original harmony. And when this harmony is restored, the geometry of the soul emerges clear, bright, luminous.

The Arcturians remind us that each human being is a forgotten song. A unique melody echoing in the stellar halls since before incarnation. Rediscovering this song is part of the ascension process. And this rediscovery happens when the being dares to listen beyond the ears, intone beyond the voice, vibrate beyond form.

The universe sings. And this song is geometry in motion. The seeker who learns to listen to this song not only understands the cosmos—they become an active part of the symphony. Each sound emitted with love is a thread of light between dimensions. And each geometry born from this sound is a bridge reconnecting the human to the divine. Sound and geometry are not separate paths. They are two sides of the same spiral. One vibrates. The other shapes. Together, they reveal the mystery. And the mystery, finally, sings its form in the awakened heart of one who remembers being light in living frequency.

Chapter 9
Codes of Light

Light contains within itself a vibrational intelligence that transcends spoken language, logical thought, and known forms. It acts as a direct link between individual consciousness and cosmic consciousness, revealing itself through patterns that are not explained, but recognized. These patterns, known as codes of light, are manifestations of the divine essence expressed in symbolic form, accessed through expanded states of perception. They carry encoded information that operates simultaneously on the spiritual, energetic, and cellular levels of the being. Each symbol is a living spark of the universal matrix, imbued with a pure intention that resonates with the stellar origin of every soul. When a code is contemplated or felt, it not only communicates an idea but activates memories, potentials, and connections that remained latent, awaiting the opportune moment to manifest.

The action of light codes does not require intellectual understanding. Their language is silent, vibrational, speaking directly to the subtle field of the being. They emerge as mandalas, fluid lines, complex geometries, or unknown characters radiating a specific vibration. When accessed, these codes align the energy field with the frequency they represent, opening channels for healing, remembrance, and reconnection. Their presence touches deep dimensions of the soul, dissolving blockages, reorganizing internal structures, and facilitating integration between the various bodies—physical, emotional, mental, and spiritual. By contemplating a code with a present heart, a process of vibrational attunement begins, allowing light to act precisely, like a key opening previously hidden doors. In this process, it is not necessary to understand the symbol with the mind, because the body, spirit, and energy field perfectly comprehend what is being transmitted.

This knowledge is cultivated and shared by high-frequency civilizations, such as the Arcturians, who operate on planes where form, sound, and light are expressions of the same primordial energy. For them, codes are not just tools—they are living consciousnesses, expressions of the very structure of the universe, destined to assist in humanity's awakening. They teach that these codes are not created, but accessed, as they already exist as part of each being's stellar memory. By coming into contact with them, the human being is not just receiving something new, but rediscovering fragments of themselves. This reconnection is transformative, as it restores alignment with the soul's mission, strengthens the connection to the source, and activates dormant gifts. Thus, codes of light reveal themselves as sacred instruments of remembrance, healing, and expansion, returning the being to its original geometry of light.

A code of light is more than a symbol—it is an energetic entity. It is generated by a specific frequency and carries within it a crystalline intention. This intention can be healing, expansion, protection, remembrance, transformation. When activated—whether by visualization, contemplation, breath, or intonation—the code emits a vibration that reorganizes the subtle fields of the being. It speaks directly to the spiritual DNA, bypassing the filters of the ego, the logical mind, and limiting beliefs. That is why its effect is often felt before being understood.

The Arcturians channel these codes in moments of vibrational alignment with the recipient's field. Often, they arise spontaneously in visions during meditation, in lucid dreams, or in creative impulses leading to automatic writing or intuitive drawing. The person doesn't understand where the symbol comes from, but feels its presence as something sacred, familiar, resonant. This happens because these codes already exist in the fabric of the spirit. The experience of channeling is, in fact, a recognition.

Each light code carries a specific geometry. Some present as spirals, others as mandalas, still others as characters resembling unknown alphabets but vibrating with unquestionable internal coherence. There are codes that activate energy centers—like the heart or pineal—and others that restructure deeper layers, such as connections with spiritual lineages, Akashic records, or the multidimensional aspects of the being.

A fundamental Arcturian practice consists of the silent contemplation of these codes. When a code is visualized with an open heart, it begins to vibrate in tune with the person's field. It acts like an antenna receiving and transmitting specific frequencies. By sustaining the gaze—not just with the eyes, but with integral presence—the practitioner allows the code to speak to their cells, their stellar memory, their mission in this incarnation. During this contemplation, subtle sensations often arise: chills, warmth in the chest, pulsations in the forehead, unexpected tears, or a deep peace enveloping the entire body. These are signs that the code is being read by the energy field and that its vibration is interacting with the being's internal system. This process does not need rational comprehension. The effect occurs even without the mind understanding. The energy field recognizes and responds.

Conscious breathing is a powerful ally in integrating the codes. By inhaling while visualizing the code and exhaling while feeling its energy spread through the body, a bridge is created between the symbol and the biological structure. The body begins to reorganize itself from that frequency. The magnetic field aligns. The spiritual DNA opens. And light begins to act as living intelligence within the being.

The Arcturians teach that there are different families of codes. There are healing codes, which act by dissolving emotional, mental, or spiritual blockages. They restore the integrity of the vibrational field and often promote immediate relief from internal pains that seemed too old to be touched. There are activation codes, which awaken latent potentials—spiritual gifts, intuitive abilities, multidimensional skills. They are like keys turning internal locks, allowing the soul to expand its range of action on this plane. There are also connection codes, which re-establish links between the incarnated being and their stellar origins. When activated, these codes open communication channels with mentors, guides, spiritual lineages, and civilizations of light. They do not impose names, doctrines, or histories—they simply vibrate. And by vibrating, they make the practitioner's field compatible with information that was previously inaccessible.

Some codes operate on collective levels. They are transmitted to harmonize groups, activate planetary networks of light, protect sacred spaces, or anchor higher frequencies in specific regions of the planet. These codes are generally channeled by souls who have a spiritual contract with Earth and who offer themselves as bridges between planes. When drawn on the ground, on the skin, or on objects, these codes radiate their vibration constantly, like subtle beacons.

The Arcturians emphasize that although light codes can be shared, their full activation depends on the recipient's vibrational state. A symbol is not magical in itself—it is a transmitter. And its effectiveness depends on attunement with the intention. By contemplating a code with presence and devotion, the practitioner activates the field it represents. But if there is distraction, doubt, or superficiality, the code remains silent. Not because it is inaccessible, but because it respects the energetic free will of each being.

The integration of codes can be deepened with intuitive vocalizations. By emitting sounds in resonance with the symbol, a toroidal field is created that envelops the practitioner and the code in a dance of light and vibration. With each chanted sound, the form intensifies. With each repetition, the light penetrates deeper. The sounds need not follow known patterns—they emerge spontaneously when the heart is open and the mind silenced.

Many spiritual artists around the world are currently channeling Arcturian codes without even consciously knowing it. Their drawings, music, dances, and words carry this vibration within them. The artist's soul recognizes the field. And the work born carries the frequency. That is why, upon observing certain arts, the seeker's heart beats stronger, eyes well up, the mind silences. The language of light is there, encoded in the forms, waiting to be decoded by the soul that recognizes it.

Creating a personal code is a transformative practice. By entering a meditative state, with a clean field and present heart, the practitioner can allow their hand to draw spontaneously. Technique or aesthetics don't matter. What emerges there is a vibrational imprint of the soul. This code can be used as a personal seal, a protection tool, an anchor of intention. It doesn't need to be understood—only felt.

The Arcturians also teach that it is possible to program crystals with these codes. By drawing or visualizing the symbol inside the crystal, and activating it with breath and sound, the crystal begins to emit that frequency continuously. It becomes a silent ally, radiating the code's vibration into the environment and the practitioner's field. This practice is used in healing chambers, sacred spaces, and ascension rituals.

Codes of light are not a language learned—they are a frequency remembered. They are present in nature, in constellations, in water patterns, in seashells, in fields of flowers. They dance in silence, waiting for the awakened gaze to rediscover them. By integrating these codes, the being returns to its origin. And upon returning, becomes a channel. Channel of light, of truth, of cosmic harmony.

Nothing more is needed. The symbol is before you. It pulses. It sings. It calls you by the name your soul knows. Simply breathe, contemplate, intone—and allow the light to reorganize you from the center to the edges of the spirit. The code is already within you. And you, now, are within it.

Chapter 10
Arcturian Healing

Arcturian healing establishes itself as a subtle and advanced science operating beyond the frontiers of dense matter, acting in the vibrational fields where dissonances originate, later manifesting as physical or emotional ailments. Unlike therapeutic approaches focusing solely on symptom elimination, this healing modality understands the being as a multidimensional unit in constant interaction with universal frequencies. Health, in this context, is not the mere absence of disease, but the reflection of internal coherence among all levels of being—physical, etheric, emotional, mental, and spiritual. When alignment exists between these bodies, vital energy flows freely, sustaining balance and vitality. The Arcturian proposal is to restore this harmony through resonance, using vibrational patterns that awaken within the individual the remembrance of their original integrity.

The healing technologies employed by the Arcturians are not based on physical instruments, but on principles of sacred geometry, conscious light, and harmonic sound, operating as catalysts for the spontaneous reorganization of the energy field. Each geometric form carries a specific code of balance; each luminous hue corresponds to an aspect of consciousness; each sound frequency touches deep layers of the being. By accessing these frequencies, whether through meditative practices or consciousness projection, the individual contacts fields of high vibrational coherence that function as multidimensional mirrors. These mirrors do not heal directly, but reflect back to the being their own capacity for regeneration, activating internal processes of self-correction and consciousness expansion. In this state of elevated resonance, blockages are dissolved, traumatic memories are reintegrated, and the soul rediscovers the path to its fullness.

This healing process is not conducted by external imposition, nor by energetic manipulation. It happens as a silent invitation from light to the light dwelling within each being. The Arcturians, by creating healing spaces on subtle planes, offer a conducive environment for realignment to occur naturally, respecting the time, frequency, and choice of each soul. Nothing is forced, everything is permitted. The individual is welcomed in their totality, without judgment, and guided to a state of deep listening where their essence can express itself freely. True healing, in this context, is a process of remembrance: remembering who one is in essence, where one came from, and the innate power of regeneration residing at the core of being. By restoring this connection with the source, the natural flow of life is re-established, and health emerges as an inevitable reflection of this reconnection.

Contrary to common perception, the Arcturians do not heal "others." They create fields that restore the internal coherence of each being. These fields, built with sacred geometry and intelligent light, act as vibrational mirrors returning to the individual the memory of their original perfection. The being's own energy field, upon recognizing this mirror, begins to reorganize spontaneously. It is in this process that healing occurs: not by external action, but by internal self-adjustment.

Arcturian healing chambers are multidimensional light structures existing on elevated planes of reality. They cannot be seen with physical eyes but are accessible through consciousness. In a deep meditative state, with the field previously prepared, it is possible to be guided to these sacred spaces. There, time is not linear, gravity does not act as on the dense plane, and energy flows in living geometric patterns. The soul is welcomed, enveloped by forms of light dancing gently around it, emitting almost imperceptible sounds that vibrate within the heart.

Each chamber is programmed to act on a specific aspect. There are chambers for cellular restoration, emotional healing, spiritual DNA alignment, vibrational reconfiguration. Upon entering one of these structures, the person's field is scanned by light entities who need not ask—they feel. There is no judgment, no diagnosis, no prognosis. There is only deep vibrational listening. The being's energy is read like an open book. And the appropriate frequencies are applied, not with invasive techniques, but with pure resonance.

These chambers are not exclusive to higher planes. It is possible to reproduce aspects of them here on Earth through conscious practices. Guided visualization is one of the most effective forms. By imagining oneself lying in a geometric structure—a golden icosahedron, a blue light dodecahedron, a circle of crystals—the practitioner creates a vibrational field simulating the Arcturian environment. By combining this visualization with conscious breathing and intonation of harmonic tones, the chamber is activated. Not by illusion, but by vibrational coherence.

Sacred geometry is essential in this process. Each form used in the chambers carries an energetic purpose. The tetrahedron stabilizes, the cube structures, the octahedron purifies, the icosahedron expands, the dodecahedron elevates. These forms, when contemplated or visualized moving around the body, generate spirals of light that dissolve blockages, deprogram limiting beliefs, and restore fluidity to the energy field. It is not about belief, but subtle physics. Form determines flow. And flow determines the state of health.

Crystals are used as amplifiers in healing sessions. Not out of superstition, but for their resonance properties. Each crystal is a vibrational antenna interacting precisely with subtle fields. Clear quartz, amethyst, selenite, blue kyanite—all possess specific signatures that, when positioned on or around the body, generate harmony. The Arcturians do not see crystals as inanimate objects, but as crystalline consciousnesses collaborating with the healing process. When programmed with light codes, these crystals become active transmitters of specific frequencies.

During an Arcturian healing session, it is common for the practitioner to feel sensations like warmth, tingling, lightness, internal pulsations, or even emotions surfacing. This occurs because the energy acts directly on the centers where there are blockages, misalignments, or unresolved traumas. Light penetrates where consciousness has not reached. And by illuminating, it reveals. This process can bring forgotten memories, old pains, or sudden revelations to the surface. All this is part of the vibrational cleansing necessary for field reorganization.

Arcturian healing does not replace earthly medicine. It complements it. It acts on levels science has yet to reach: the subtle bodies. Many physical illnesses are just the final stage of imbalances that began in the energetic and emotional bodies. Treating only the physical symptom leaves the pattern intact. But by treating the field, the root is dissolved. And the body responds with balance.

Self-healing is one of the central pillars of Arcturian teaching. Every being possesses the innate ability to restore their harmony. The Arcturians do not wish to create dependence, but spiritual autonomy. Therefore, they teach practices anyone can apply in daily life. Contemplating mandalas, meditating with geometries, intuitive use of crystals, vocalizing specific tones, vibrational programming of water—all are accessible paths to maintain the field in a state of flow and integrity.

Water, in particular, is an extraordinary vehicle for healing. When exposed to geometric forms, colors, sounds, and elevated intentions, it absorbs these frequencies and transmits them to the body upon ingestion. Water is a vibrational mirror. Programming it with an Arcturian code, activated by vocalization and light, transforms it into a vibrational elixir. This simple gesture can profoundly alter deeply ingrained internal patterns. The Arcturians use water in rituals of vibrational restoration, always with gratitude and reverence, recognizing its sacred intelligence.

Another powerful practice is projecting consciousness to healing chambers during sleep. Before falling asleep, by clearly stating the intention and surrendering to the Arcturian presence with trust, the being is guided, in subtle body, to the spaces of light where necessary adjustments are made. Upon awakening, even if nothing is remembered, the body feels it: there is lightness, clarity, peace. The field has been touched, and something has reorganized.

It is fundamental to remember that each healing process is unique. What works for one may not resonate with another. The Arcturians respect this singularity. They do not standardize—they personalize. The soul's frequency is the compass. And the healing journey is always conducted with unconditional love. There is never imposition. Only invitation. Light is always available, but it is the being who decides when to open to it.

Healing, for the Arcturians, is remembrance. Remembering that there was never separation. That imbalance is a temporary disconnection from the source of light. And that by reconnecting, everything returns to its natural state of harmony. It is not magic. It is remembrance. And upon remembering, the body, mind, spirit, and soul return to dancing in unison the sacred music of the universe.

The field of healing already pulses around. The light already calls the soul's name. And the heart, upon silencing, knows: healing does not come from outside. It emerges from the center. And the center, now, shines with the frequency of Arcturus.

Chapter 11
Flower of Life

The Flower of Life manifests as the primordial pattern sustaining all creation, a vibrational matrix that precedes any language, dogma, or conceptual limitation. It represents the structural intelligence of the universe, a sacred code imprinted on the very essence of spacetime. Its presence is not symbolic but functional: it acts as the invisible foundation upon which all forms organize themselves, from the smallest subatomic particles to the vastest galaxies. The Arcturians, with their expanded consciousness and multidimensional perception, recognize in the Flower of Life the direct emanation of the Source, the original architecture that anchors unity amidst diversity.

In their studies and practices, this geometry is not merely observed but experienced as a living organism, capable of interacting with the subtlest levels of being. When one accesses the vibration of the Flower of Life, something profound is activated at the core of the being: a silent remembrance, prior to earthly experiences, echoing directly from stellar memory. This remembrance occurs not through logical reasoning, but through direct resonance with the field the Flower emits. Its intertwined circles, composed with mathematical precision, form a field of coherence that acts as a bridge between the conscious and the superconscious. The energy emanating from it organizes internal chaos, repositions fragments of multidimensional identity, and re-establishes the flow between the incarnated being and their Higher Self.

The Flower of Life is not just visually harmonious—it is a transmitter of cosmic order, a silent language speaking directly to the spiritual DNA. Interaction with this sacred geometry, whether through contemplation, meditation, or manual reproduction, initiates an alchemical process in the subtle field. When drawing it, the practitioner performs not just an aesthetic activity, but contacts the vibrational pattern of the universe. Each stroke is a conscious gesture repositioning the being in relation to the Source. The Arcturians teach that by engaging with the Flower of Life, the personal energy field aligns with the universal rhythm, facilitating healing, consciousness expansion, and access to elevated planes of reality. This pattern, when activated in the body, becomes a nucleus of intelligent light, radiating harmony to the chakras, organs, and cells. Thus, the Flower of Life fulfills its original role: reconnecting each being to their divine origin, restoring the natural state of fullness and unity with the whole.

The Flower of Life is composed of multiple circles intertwined with mathematical precision, forming a field of absolute symmetry. Looking at it is like contemplating God's plan. Each circle is a note in the score of existence. And their intertwining creates harmony, proportion, rhythm, resonance. It does not merely represent creation—it contains it. It is present in DNA, in shells, in galaxies, in flower petals, in sacred architecture, and in the light temples of interdimensional civilizations. Where life pulses, the Flower of Life vibrates.

For the Arcturians, this structure is not just a symbol; it is a living tool for communication between planes. Each intersection of its circles acts as an activation point. By contemplating the Flower of Life with presence, the observer's energy field begins to resonate with its frequency. This simple act awakens cosmic memories, activates latent codes in the spiritual DNA, and expands perception beyond the limits of the linear mind.

The practice of drawing the Flower of Life is considered a sacred exercise. It is not just geometric art—it is active meditation, a process of alignment between the microcosm and the macrocosm. The Arcturians teach that by tracing the circles with intention, the being inscribes the pattern of creation into space. The pencil becomes a conductor of light. The hand, an extension of the soul. And the paper, a projection of the vibrational field undergoing reorganization. Each stroke is a thread connecting the visible to the invisible. Upon completing the first rosette—formed by seven intertwined circles—the field already begins to pulse. It is as if a vibrational mandala emerges from the two-dimensional plane and starts radiating energy in all directions. This initial configuration is known as the Seed of Life. It contains the essence of creation, the principle of everything. When expanded, this seed blossoms. And upon blossoming, it reveals the Flower.

Contemplating this geometry has profound effects. By fixing the eyes—and especially the heart—on the Flower of Life, one begins to perceive subtle changes in the field. Thoughts slow down. Dense emotions dissolve. Sensations of expansion, openness in the chest center, and lightness in the physical body become frequent. This occurs because the Flower of Life emits a frequency of coherence. It acts like a spiritual tuning fork, restoring alignment between the subtle bodies and the soul's original matrix.

In Arcturian temples, the Flower of Life is present in almost all structures. Not for decoration, but for function. The walls vibrate with this pattern. The ceilings, altars, crystals used in rituals—everything is imbued with this geometry. It is used as a basis for programming healing chambers, constructing protective fields, activating light-ships, and for interdimensional teaching. Where the Flower of Life is present, there is order, harmony, and flow.

The Arcturians also transmit variations of this form, known as Stellar Flowers. These are expansions of the original geometry that include additional codes intended for souls operating on specific missions. These variations might contain more circles, fractal structures, interconnected stars, or internal spirals. Each is designed for a purpose: healing, teaching, interdimensional travel, cellular reconfiguration, communication with other realities. Upon receiving these flowers, the being is invited to integrate forgotten aspects of their cosmic mission.

One of the most notable aspects of the Flower of Life is its ability to awaken cosmic memory. By interacting with it—whether through contemplation, drawing, or meditation—the practitioner begins to access records beyond the reach of the conscious mind. Vivid dreams, spontaneous visions, sensations of deep recognition, images of stellar civilizations, or memories of past lives in elevated worlds become more frequent. This happens because the Flower's geometry acts as a master key in the vibrational field, unlocking the inner doors of knowing.

The practice of meditating with the Flower of Life involves more than looking at it. It involves breathing with it. Inhaling as if the air comes from the intersections of its circles. Exhaling as if light emanates from its center. With each breath, the field expands. The geometry begins to spin, not just on the visual plane, but within the being's energy field. The Flower becomes alive, pulsating, and the practitioner, one with its vibration.

It is also possible to activate the Flower of Life on the body itself. Visualize it spinning in the center of the chest, its light expanding with each heartbeat. Feel its circles touching the lungs, diaphragm, spine. Allow it to become the core of your field. Then, visualize it beneath the feet, above the head, in the energy centers. This multidimensional field of energetic blossoming generates protection, cleansing, and elevation.

Crystals engraved with the Flower of Life have properties of vibrational amplification. They can be used in rituals, meditations, or simply placed in sacred spaces. When activated with light and intention, they become continuous transmitters of harmony. Water can be programmed with the Flower. By placing a symbol under a glass of water for a few hours, the water's molecular structure begins to reflect the geometric patterns, transforming it into an elixir of cellular reorganization.

At certain planetary moments, like solstices, equinoxes, and numerical portals, the energy of the Flower of Life intensifies. The Arcturians advise that on these days, practices with this geometry become even more potent. It is as if the cosmos opens direct channels to the universal matrix, and the Flower acts as a perfect intermediary between the plane of form and the plane of spirit.

In Arcturian schools, the Flower of Life is taught from the earliest levels of initiation. Each student learns not only to draw it but to feel it. They learn to navigate its layers, decipher its codes, use it as a light-ship. For when fully activated, the Flower of Life is not just a mandala—it is a portal. A transition point between worlds. A unified field leading the being from fragmentation to unity.

Looking at the Flower of Life is contemplating the mirror of one's own soul. Seeing it awakens something. Something returns. Something remembers. And in this remembering, there is no effort, no pain, no searching. There is only presence. The being breathes, the Flower pulses. And creation, in silence, blossoms again in the center of the chest. The Flower of Life is the mother of all forms. The sacred womb where light bends into beauty. And when the being unites with it, there is no longer separation between creator and creation. There is only the dance. The dance of eternal geometry singing the forgotten language of perfection. And whoever hears, whoever sees, whoever feels—is never the same again. Because they no longer walk the line of time, but the spiral of remembrance. The spiral of life. The spiral of the flower that never ceased to bloom.

Chapter 12
Golden Ratio

The Golden Ratio manifests as a universal principle governing the intrinsic harmony of the cosmos, reflecting the organizing intelligence of life in all its expressions. This mathematical ratio, expressed by the constant 1.618..., appears not just as a numerical curiosity or a tool for aesthetic composition, but as a subtle and constant presence in the fundamental structures of reality. Its action is not restricted to the physical or visible plane—it traverses dimensions and inscribes itself onto the very vibrational fabric of existence. Wherever the flow of creation moves with balance, precision, and beauty, this proportion is present, guiding the development of forms with a pattern that precedes and transcends rational consciousness. It need not be discovered, as it is already imprinted on everything true, coherent, and alive. Life, in its essence, organizes itself from this matrix of silent order.

In the understanding of the Arcturians, this proportion is a primordial language of the Source—a code of light translating into forms, sounds, movements, and frequencies. What the eyes recognize as beautiful and harmonious, the integral being experiences as resonance with the very matrix of the universe. Beauty, in this context, is not an external attribute, but a vibration aligning the being with its origin. When a structure—be it a flower, a temple, a galactic spiral, or an artistic composition—follows the Golden Ratio, it acts as a mirror of the creative consciousness, awakening in the observer an ancestral memory of order, belonging, and unity. This memory is not stored in the logical mind, but inscribed in the subtle fields of the being, accessible only through vibrational sensitivity.

By understanding and applying the Golden Ratio, the Arcturians seek not just to replicate nature's aesthetics, but to create fields of coherence that re-establish communication with the original flow of life. In their wisdom, every mandala, architectural structure, emitted sound, or sacred gesture is imbued with this proportion, aiming to generate environments and experiences that favor the being's energetic reorganization. This reorganization is not imposed—it is awakened. For the Golden Ratio acts as a silent reminder, an inner compass guiding the being back to the center, where the soul's frequency finds its purest expression. Thus, the presence of this proportion is more than a mathematical manifestation: it is the living signature of cosmic perfection in motion.

The Golden Ratio, or golden number, represents a ratio between parts that repeats in nature with absolute perfection. Expressed numerically as 1.618..., its presence is constant: in the spiral of galaxies, the arrangement of flower petals, the structure of DNA, the growth of shells, human anatomy, facial proportions, river curves, ocean waves. Wherever life organizes itself with fluidity and beauty, there it is—silent, precise, eternal.

For the Arcturians, this proportion is not merely an expression of aesthetics, but a vibrational frequency. What the human mind perceives as beautiful, harmonious, and pleasing to the eye is, in fact, a reflection of the vibrational coherence of light in its material manifestation. Beauty is not a judgment—it is an unconscious recognition of the presence of divine order. When something resonates with the Golden Ratio, it also resonates with the original field of creation. The being feels this, even without rational understanding.

This recognition is not just contemplative—it is functional. Upon contacting forms expressing the golden ratio, the human energy field begins to reorganize. The mind quiets. Emotions stabilize. The body aligns. This happens because the golden ratio communicates to the vibrational field an archetypal model of balance. It is as if it says: "this is the natural flow of light." And the field, upon listening, begins to remember.

In Arcturian practices, the Golden Ratio is used as the basis for constructing mandalas, healing structures, dimensional portals, and chambers for energetic regeneration. Every angle, distance, curve is calculated to resonate with this proportion. Upon entering these spaces—physical or subtle—the being is enveloped by a vibrational mesh of pure order. This envelopment does not force transformation. It invites surrender. And by surrendering, the being restructures.

The Arcturians teach that the human body, when viewed with initiated eyes, is a sacred temple built upon the golden geometry. The proportions between bones, organ placement, hand shape, heartbeat rhythm—all respond to this pattern. When the body sickens, what occurs is a departure from this harmony. And when it returns to proportion, health flourishes. Healing, therefore, is a vibrational remembrance of the geometry of light.

Meditating with the golden spiral is a profoundly transformative practice. The spiral, growing according to the Fibonacci sequence—a progression approaching the golden ratio—is the most natural form of expansion in the universe. From hurricanes to galaxies, it is the path of energy moving in ordered expansion. By visualizing it during meditation, spiraling outward from the chest center, the practitioner activates this frequency in the energy field. This spiral can be visualized as a path of golden light spinning slowly, expanding with each breath. As the spiral grows, it traverses the energy centers, aligning them, awakening cosmic memories, dissolving blockages. The golden spiral does not force opening—it invites the field to flow. And in flow, there is no resistance.

The Fibonacci sequence—1, 1, 2, 3, 5, 8, 13, 21, 34, 55...—is another way to integrate the golden frequency into consciousness. Each number in the sequence is the sum of the two preceding it. This progression, manifesting in countless natural forms, is also a vibrational code. By vocalizing the numbers with intention, or chanting mantras whose syllables follow this progression (as in rhythmic series of tones), a resonant field is created that attracts cosmic order. Musical instruments tuned based on the 432 Hz frequency, for example, resonate more closely with the Golden Ratio than those tuned to the standard 440 Hz frequency. The Arcturians use sounds following this harmony to adjust the subtle fields of beings in transition. Music becomes a vibrational bridge between internal chaos and universal order. Upon listening, the being is touched on levels words cannot reach.

Sacred architecture is also based on the Golden Ratio. Ancient Egyptians, Greeks, Renaissance artists, Templar masters, the Vedas of India—all used this proportion to erect temples that were not just physical spaces, but frequency structures. When the body enters a space built on this pattern, it feels welcomed, protected, elevated. This is not illusion—it is resonance. The Arcturians, in their ships and cities of light, build everything from this proportion. This is what keeps their fields stable, light, integrated with higher consciousness.

The presence of the Golden Ratio in nature is not random. Each leaf, flower, living structure grows to reflect this flow. This is because Earth's own consciousness is imbued with this pattern. By walking through forests, observing the sea, contemplating mountains and animals, the being can absorb this frequency simply through mindful attention. That is why so many feel healing when in contact with nature: it vibrates with the harmony the human mind has lost, but the heart still remembers.

Art is another channel for expressing this divine geometry. Paintings, sculptures, photographs, even dances—when created under the inspiration of the Golden Ratio, become transmitters of balance. The eyes scan the work, the body responds, the mind silences. There is no explanation—only sensation. Art vibrates, and by vibrating, communicates. The Arcturians encourage artists to reconnect with this frequency, allowing creation to be more than aesthetics: to be vibrational medicine.

Activating the body through the Golden Ratio can also be done with gestures. Certain movements, when executed according to angles and curves compatible with this proportion, generate toroidal fields of light around the practitioner. These gestures, combined with breath and visualization, become a form of geometry in motion. It is like dancing the structure of the cosmos. And by dancing, the being becomes one with the dance of creation.

The Arcturians state that the Golden Ratio is not just a pattern of form—it is a frequency of the soul. When the being vibrates in this proportion, they feel at home. Everything flows. Decisions become clear. Relationships balance. The body responds with lightness. Intuition intensifies. Not because everything is "solved," but because everything is in flow. And where there is flow, there is true life. This is the silent beauty of the Golden Ratio: it does not impose, demand, or shout. It simply is. It always has been. And when the being begins to perceive it within, around, and in all living things, they return to their own primordial structure. Not as an idea—but as embodied vibration.

The path reveals itself in spirals. And in each turn of the spiral, the being rediscovers themselves with new eyes. The Golden Ratio does not lead to a destination—it leads to the center. And in the center, where there is no time, form, or name, pulses the geometric heart of the Source. The same that breathes in you. The same that now reminds you: you are made of light in perfect order.

Chapter 13
Platonic Solids

Five perfect forms sustain, in their structure and frequency, the invisible pillars of material and spiritual existence. They not only compose the basis of three-dimensional geometry but also organize, guide, and manifest fundamental patterns of the universe. These forms, known as the Platonic Solids, do not emerge by chance but reflect a primordial intelligence governing everything from the smallest subatomic particles to the largest galaxies. Their essence surpasses the field of mathematics and inserts itself deeply into the core of humanity's most ancient spiritual traditions. They are patterns vibrating with such precision that they become languages, capable of translating universal harmony into structure, movement, and consciousness.

These solids express universal archetypal principles transcending cultures and epochs, acting as activation keys revealing the symmetry between the visible and the invisible. Each of these geometric forms carries a unique vibrational field resonating with natural elements and subtle aspects of human and cosmic experience. When studied or contemplated deeply, they reveal encoded wisdom, ancestral knowledge continuing to echo in teachings left by civilizations like Atlantis, Ancient Egypt, and Eastern mystical lineages.

The Arcturians, beings of elevated consciousness, recognize in these solids the living structure of creation. For them, they are not just geometric figures, but conscious entities organizing light into forms, energy into direction, and consciousness into purpose. By using these solids as meditative and structural tools, these beings establish bridges between planes of existence, accessing realities where linear thought gives way to the fractal perception of unity. Contact with these forms, therefore, is more than symbolic or decorative. It is an experience of reconnection with the original matrix of existence. Tetrahedron, cube, octahedron, dodecahedron, and icosahedron are more than geometric elements—they are molds of light in its cosmic dance. When activated in conscious practices, these solids act as catalysts for transformation, realigning subtle bodies and awakening expanded states of perception. Therefore, the Arcturians consider them silent masters: guardians of wisdoms that are not spoken, but felt and become. In this context, understanding the Platonic Solids is more than learning about shapes. It is remembering, on a cellular and spiritual level, the original language with which the universe sings its own existence.

Plato described them in Ancient Greece, but he did not invent them. He rediscovered them, like many before and after him. In esoteric schools of Atlantis, in pre-dynastic Egypt, in pyramid chambers, in Toltec and Vedic traditions, these solids were always used as tools of wisdom and transmutation. Their power lies not just in their symmetry, but in their coherence with the matrix of light.

There are five: tetrahedron, cube, octahedron, dodecahedron, and icosahedron. Together, they form the backbone of three-dimensional sacred geometry.

The tetrahedron, with its four triangular faces, is the symbol of fire. It represents action, transformation, spiritual will. Its vertices point in all directions of existence, and its shape creates stability with a minimum number of faces. It is a sharp, penetrating body that stimulates the ascensional movement of consciousness. In Arcturian meditations, the tetrahedron is used to activate the solar plexus and catalyze processes of internal transmutation. When mentally rotated in the field, it burns old patterns and makes space for renewed light.

The cube, composed of six square faces, is the solid of earth. It symbolizes stability, manifestation, and the physical body. Its form evokes foundation, the structure that sustains. The Arcturians use it to anchor elevated frequencies in physical environments. By visualizing a cube of light under the feet, the practitioner establishes a connection with Earth's energy grid. This cube is also known as "Gaia's Cube"—a vibrational container protecting and stabilizing the energy field of beings undergoing ascension.

The octahedron, with its eight triangular faces, is linked to air. It is a symbol of integration, the flow between the higher and lower. With one vertex pointing to the sky and another to the earth, the octahedron is the axis between planes. In Arcturian practices, it is positioned around the heart, creating a field of loving neutrality. This field allows the welcoming of polarity without judgment. It is a crystalline mirror where light and shadow can coexist, dialogue, reconcile.

The dodecahedron, with its twelve pentagonal faces, is the body of ether—the subtlest element, invisible, yet present in everything. It is linked to spirit, consciousness expansion, and connection to the unified field. When the dodecahedron spins around the head during meditations, the pineal gland is activated, inner vision expands, and the mind attunes to multidimensional frequencies. The Arcturians use this solid in teaching chambers, where information is transmitted not by words, but by resonance.

The icosahedron, with its twenty triangular faces, represents water. It is a symbol of fluidity, emotional healing, adaptability. Spinning around the emotional body, it dissolves patterns of pain and opens channels for true feeling. In regeneration practices, the Arcturians envelop the practitioner's field with translucent icosahedrons vibrating in shades of blue and green, emitting codes that restore emotional integrity. Water, like the icosahedron, always finds the path. Always returns to its source.

Each of these solids fits perfectly inside a sphere, and all share unique characteristics: congruent faces, identical angles, perfect symmetry. Therefore, they are considered "Platonic"—pure, ideal. But for the Arcturians, their value resides not in formal perfection. It resides in the frequency they emit. Each form is a note in the chord of creation. By combining these forms in geometric practices, the being begins to compose their own vibrational melody.

Working with the Platonic Solids is not just contemplative—it is transformative. By visualizing each form in meditation, placed upon, within, or around the body, a process of vibrational resonance begins. The field responds. Chakras align. Subtle bodies organize. Not by imposition, but by coherence. The pattern enters and disorder yields. Light reorganizes itself.

Arcturian practices involve the sequential use of these solids. First, the cube, to stabilize the field. Then, the icosahedron, to release emotions. Next, the octahedron, to integrate. The tetrahedron, then, activates will. And the dodecahedron, finally, expands consciousness. Each session is unique but follows this fluid logic of energetic construction. There is no rush. Each form remains in conscious rotation for a few minutes. The effects are subtle but profound: mental clarity, emotional lightness, alignment with purpose.

The solids can also be physically arranged in the environment, as carved crystals or geometric forms built with natural materials. When positioned in specific patterns—like the five-pointed star, circle, or spiral—they create fields of protection, activation, or teaching. These arrangements, called structural mandalas, act as vibrational devices transforming any space into a sacred environment.

Besides meditative practices, it's possible to use the solids in directed visualizations. For example, when facing conflict, one can envelop the situation in an octahedron of silver light, allowing opposites to balance. When seeking clarity for a decision, one can invoke the golden dodecahedron above the head. In moments of instability, the cube under the feet grounds and restores. These simple gestures reprogram the field in real-time.

Arcturian ships, often reported as floating geometric structures, are built based on the Platonic solids and their multidimensional variations. They have no screws or engines. They are fields of condensed light, programmed with sacred geometry, reacting to the consciousness of those inhabiting them. These ships are extensions of the being—not means of transport, but of manifestation. Where the being vibrates in coherence, the ship forms.

The Platonic Solids are not just forms of space—they are forms of spirit. Each contains a key to awakening. By interacting with these forms, the being begins to remember forgotten aspects of their own nature. Begins to see themselves no longer as a body in a world, but as a light field in a network of divine patterns. This perception is not philosophical—it is vibrational.

The geometric awakening these forms provide is silent but irreversible. Once the being vibrates with the dodecahedron, for example, their consciousness no longer returns to linearity. It expands spirally, recognizing in nature's forms the reflection of its own essence. Each leaf, crystal, cell becomes a mirror of origin.

The Arcturians invite each soul to explore these forms with reverence, not as objects, but as masters. The cube teaches rooting. The tetrahedron, action. The octahedron, integration. The icosahedron, flow. The dodecahedron, transcendence. And together, these five bodies build the bridge between the visible and the invisible, between the human and the cosmic. The inner temple rises from these forms. Light bends over them. Spirit dances in them. And by walking through this living geometry, the being recognizes: they were always made of forms that sing. And this song, now, leads them back to the home they never left—the sacred center of creation.

Chapter 14
Cosmic Toroid

At the core of the universal structure, an organizing principle manifests that transcends the linear understanding of reality: a dynamic, self-regulating, interconnected energy matrix constituting the essence of all existence. This matrix reveals itself in a precise and recurring geometric form—the toroid—whose presence extends from the smallest particles to the largest celestial bodies. It is a living, pulsating energetic architecture expressing the perennial cycle of vital flow: energy emerges from the center, expands in all directions, curves at the periphery, and returns to the origin point, completing a continuous feedback loop. This universal pulsation not only sustains the functioning of matter but also reflects a principle of consciousness in motion, structuring how life manifests, evolves, and interacts on all planes of being.

The nature of the cosmic toroid is not merely a conceptual abstraction or a symbolic visual construction; it is an observable energetic reality in electromagnetic fields, nature's growth patterns, and the regeneration mechanisms of body and soul. Its spiraled logic mirrors how light travels, planets orbit, branches unfold, chakras spin. This configuration reveals that everything is in constant renewal, and nothing remains static. By understanding this structure as the foundation of the manifest universe, it becomes evident that every being, atom, and thought is inserted into a system of constant exchange—a cosmic breath where there is no beginning or end, only transformation. Energy, circulating in this format, does not dissipate but recycles and elevates in complexity and consciousness, offering the being the opportunity to align with the primordial flow of creation.

Thus, recognizing the toroid as the foundation of existence is also recognizing oneself as an inseparable part of an intelligent and vibrant whole. This awakens in the human being the memory that their personal energy is not isolated or limited to the physical body's boundaries but resonates with a larger field that informs, nourishes, and responds to their internal frequency. When the being's center aligns with this universal geometry, a new perception is born: that reality is shaped by coherent vibrational patterns, and inner balance generates outer harmony. From this consciousness, it becomes possible to understand that spirituality is not separate from science, the invisible sustains the visible, and the key to awakening lies in recognizing one's own body and field as living mirrors of the universe in flow. At this point of convergence, the toroid is not just a form—it is the path.

The toroid is a sacred geometric structure representing the infinite cycle of energy in motion. Visually, it can be compared to a three-dimensional doughnut, but its complexity goes far beyond what eyes can perceive. Its center is a convergence point where energy collapses to be reborn in continuous flow. Everything living vibrates in this pattern. Breathing follows the toroidal flow. The human heart's electromagnetic field pulses in this geometry. Earth's energy, with its poles and force lines, does too.

For the Arcturians, the toroid is more than a form: it is the structure of consciousness in motion. When light decides to manifest, it spins. And by spinning, it creates a self-feeding field. This field is self-sustaining, intelligent, and responds to intention. Every being awakening to their true nature begins to perceive this pattern within themselves. Vital energy doesn't come from outside. It is generated at the very center. And the center is in everything.

Understanding the toroid is a key to reconnection. When the being starts perceiving themselves as a toroidal field of light, they abandon the idea of separation. They are no longer an isolated body in the world, but a point of convergence and emission, in constant exchange with the whole. The energy entering and leaving their heart center, chakras, consciousness, is not lost—it circulates, returns, transforms. In this flow, there is no waste. There is learning.

Activating the personal toroid is initiating the process of vibrational self-sustainment. This means stopping seeking vital force externally—in people, events, ideas—and starting to generate, through intention, breath, and expanded consciousness, one's own flow. When this occurs, the being becomes a radiant center. Their actions emanate coherence. Their field attracts harmony. Their thoughts align with the cosmos's matrix. They do not depend—they interact.

The human heart's toroidal field is one of the most beautiful examples of this dynamic. Scientists have proven the heart emits a much more potent electromagnetic field than the brain. This field extends meters from the body and responds to emotions, thoughts, states of presence. When the being enters a state of gratitude, love, or contemplation, this field expands and assumes a more coherent, luminous, powerful toroidal shape.

The Arcturians use the toroid as the basis for all their light technologies. Their ships, for example, do not function with linear propulsion. They operate by toroidal fields that bend space around them, allowing interdimensional displacement without continuity rupture. The ship doesn't "move" in the earthly sense—it reorganizes the surrounding field until the new position is reached by vibrational convergence. This is only possible because the consciousness aboard sustains the toroid's coherence.

In healing chambers, the toroid is used to envelop the being in a field of constant regeneration. The symbol is visualized, activated with geometry and sound, and sustained by crystals and lights spinning at specific rhythms. Upon entering this field, the practitioner's energy body begins to reorganize. Pain patterns are dissolved at the toroid's center and recycled at the edge, returning as purified light. Healing is not imposed—it results from the flow's intelligence.

A fundamental Arcturian practice for personal toroid activation involves conscious breathing combined with visualization. The practitioner sits silently, aligns the spine, relaxes the body. Upon inhaling, visualizes energy rising from Earth's center through the body's central axis, passing through all chakras, exiting the crown. Upon exhaling, energy returns from the cosmos, descends the same axis, re-entering Earth. This continuous flow creates a toroidal spiral around the body, expanding more with each breath. As the practice deepens, the field intensifies. This flow can be visualized as a golden, blue, or violet light spiral, gently spinning around the body, from center outward, top to bottom, in all directions. Over time, this field becomes perceptible even to subtle touch. Sensations of warmth, tingling, lightness, expansion become common. The practitioner is not just meditating—they are navigating.

This toroidal field can be programmed with intention. The Arcturians teach that by declaring, with presence and truth, an intention for healing, protection, expansion, or learning, the personal toroid absorbs this information and propagates it spirally. Intention doesn't disperse—it circulates. And by circulating, it strengthens, refines, manifests. The toroid is a creation field. It transforms thought into form, emotion into reality, vibration into experience.

The toroid is also the basis for interdimensional communication. By attuning the field with the universal toroid—the consciousness mesh interconnecting all beings—it becomes possible to receive information from higher planes, spiritual guides, stellar civilizations.

This attunement requires not mental effort, but inner silence and coherent heart frequency. It is at the toroid's center, where everything collapses into a point, that subtle listening occurs. There is no noise, no words. Only pure vibration. And this vibration is living language.

The toroid's geometry appears in various sacred traditions. It's implicit in chakra structures, ancient labyrinths, Tibetan mandalas, Gothic cathedral tracery. It's also in crop circles, shell spirals, hurricane patterns. Nature, in its silent intelligence, builds everything from this flow. Where there is true life, there is a toroid.

Each chakra, when activated, spins in a toroidal spiral. Each cell, upon receiving coherent light, reorganizes in this pattern. The human aura, when fully expanded, takes the form of a multi-layered toroid. The soul, connecting with its higher versions, creates interconnected toroidal fields keeping it stable during expansion.

The Arcturians state that humanity's next evolutionary leap is linked to toroid consciousness. When humans understand themselves as fields in flow—not bodies in conflict—planetary healing will happen rapidly. Disease, fear, scarcity, separation result from collapsed, fragmented, disorganized fields. Restoring flow restores life.

Therefore, cultivating the personal toroid is an act of service to light. Each being sustaining their field with coherence, intention, love, affects the network of all others. Light circulating in a conscious field reaches places words cannot. And by touching, transforms. By spinning, heals. By returning, teaches.

The toroid need not be understood—only experienced. It is within you. Breathe. Silence. Feel. At your being's center, there's a spinning point of light. This light is your origin. This spin is your path. And the flow, now awakened, already begins to sing your name in creation's eternal choir.

Chapter 15
Metatron's Cube

There exists a geometric structure whose presence transcends the symbolic field and enters the domains of active consciousness, functioning as a direct mechanism for spiritual alignment and vibrational expansion. This is Metatron's Cube, a formation synthesizing universal principles into a living architecture, acting as an instrument for reconnection with the higher intelligences of the cosmos. This sacred geometry not only represents the intrinsic harmony of the universe—it manifests, emits, and establishes it around whoever accesses it. In its essence, Metatron's Cube is not just an encoded drawing: it pulses with the original frequency of Creation, serving as a catalyst for elevating perception, activating spiritual memory, and realigning with the subtlest states of multidimensional reality. Its action is not passive, nor merely contemplative; rather, it is an intelligent, conscious, responsive field, acting as a bridge between the human and the divine, between the visible and the invisible.

The formation of Metatron's Cube arises as a natural expansion of the Flower of Life, unfolding into a structure containing all fundamental principles of sacred geometry, housing the five Platonic Solids, and revealing the underlying fabric of Creation. Each point, line, intersection possesses a specific resonance, capable of interacting with the various levels of being—physical, emotional, mental, spiritual. In this cohesive geometric field, everything vibrates in order and coherence. The Cube's presence can dissolve chaotic patterns, restore energetic balance, and reconfigure the vibrational mesh connecting the individual to their original purpose.

For advanced civilizations like the Arcturians, it is more than a symbol: it is an active tool for healing, teaching, elevation, used in transmutation rituals and light chambers dedicated to conscious awakening. When integrated into visualization, meditation, or energetic encoding practices, Metatron's Cube becomes an agent of profound transformation, awakening the remembrance of the divine within the being. It activates cellular intelligence, reorganizes genetic information, creates a direct bridge to the Akashic Records, facilitating access to higher levels of wisdom. Its action is not limited to the practitioner's interiority—it reverberates into the surrounding reality, refining links with time, space, matter. Everything begins aligning with a subtler order, where intentions become more precise, encounters more significant, life's movements more synchronous. The Cube is not just an instrument for spiritual contemplation; it is an encoded light body, an activation channel that, once accessed, transforms the being's field into a mirror of cosmic harmony.

Metatron's Cube is born from the Flower of Life. When the thirteen fundamental circles are extracted from its core and each center connected with straight lines, this figure pulsing with divine energy is obtained. At the Cube's center rest the five Platonic Solids, revealing the perfect integration between all elements of creation: fire, water, earth, air, ether. This alone makes the Cube a bridge between the material world and the realms of pure consciousness.

For the Arcturians, Metatron's Cube is a conscious field. It doesn't just represent harmony—it emits harmony. Doesn't just symbolize balance—it generates balance. When activated with presence, sound, light, this field expands around the practitioner, creating a living geometric mesh restructuring subtle bodies. Disordered mental patterns begin dissolving. Emotional blockages lose strength. Spiritual memories realign with their original vibration.

Metatron, as an entity, is known as the cosmic architect, guardian of universal records, link between the human world and angelic spheres of wisdom. The Arcturians collaborate with this intelligence, recognizing him as an ambassador of universal harmony. The Cube bearing his name is the geometric form through which this consciousness operates. It is not just a symbol attributed to a being—it is the vibrational body of a cosmic consciousness in active form.

By contemplating Metatron's Cube, the being starts attuning to its internal architecture. Each line, intersection, angle acts as a frequency touching specific aspects of the energy field. Simple contemplation of this symbol already initiates vibrational cleansing. But when allied with guided visualization and meditation practices, the Cube transforms into an ascension vehicle.

A fundamental Arcturian practice involves visualizing the Cube spinning slowly over the practitioner's field. First, positioned above the head, like a geometric light crown. Spinning clockwise, it begins emanating a golden spiral penetrating through the crown center. Light travels down the spine, touches each chakra, awakens dormant centers. Upon reaching the base of the spine, the Cube is then visualized spinning oppositely, bringing light back upwards, unifying vital energy poles. This double movement—top-down and bottom-up—activates the toroidal flow within the human field. And since the Cube contains all geometric elements of creation, this flow not only expands but orders. Consciousness clears. Perception opens. The sensation is of entering a subtler spacetime, where everything vibrates in a harmony the mind could never construct alone.

Metatron's Cube is also an instrument of vibrational protection. The Arcturians use it to create energetic shielding fields around beings in moments of expansion, transition, vulnerability. Visualized in continuous rotation around the body, it forms a vibrational matrix preventing dissonant frequency entry. But this shield isn't rigid. It's intelligent. It filters, rather than blocks. Allows light in, repels distortions.

Furthermore, the Cube is used as a tool for accessing Akashic Records. Activated in deep meditation, it positions itself at the center of the higher mind—a subtle region of consciousness located above the crown chakra. From this point, it emits patterns aligning the being's frequency with higher layers of the cosmic informational field. It is in this state that visions, words, images, sensations of knowing not learned but recalled begin emerging. The Cube doesn't reveal content—it opens the door for the soul itself to recognize.

Crystals programmed with Metatron's Cube become powerful transmitters. The Arcturians use crystalline spheres and prisms engraved with this pattern in their teaching and healing chambers. Positioned at specific field points, these crystals amplify the Cube's geometry, generating holographic fields reorganizing even vibrational patterns of cellular structure. Healing happens not just ethereally—it descends to DNA, to the cell nucleus, reorganizing information sustaining health and consciousness.

The Cube can also be physically drawn and used as a meditative mandala. The simple act of tracing it with intention is already a practice of presence and connection. Each drawn line is an emanation of light in the invisible mesh connecting the practitioner to the Arcturian field. Upon completion, the Cube becomes a geometric altar. It can be used as a base for rituals, crystal activation, water programming, attunement with guides, perception expansion.

In Arcturian light schools, Metatron's Cube is one of the first symbols given to initiates. Not as an object of worship, but as a map. A map pointing not to a location, but a state of being. It teaches through silence. Each rotation is a lesson. Each intersection, a meeting point between dimensions. Each edge, a path. And each form within it, a living frequency, awaiting to be felt.

By working with the Cube, the being starts perceiving changes not only in their energy field but also in their external reality. Disharmonious situations begin dissolving. Synchronicities increase. Time becomes more fluid. Words gain weight, thoughts direction. This is because the Cube acts not just as a meditation tool—it reprograms the relationship between the being and the universe. Aligns intentions. Refines desires. Harmonizes actions.

Metatron's Cube is not a hidden secret for a few. It is a universal gift, a response from the Source to those seeking to remember who they are. It is available, accessible, present in all cultures that touched the sacred light. And now, with the planetary awakening underway, it re-emerges as a silent guide—not to be venerated, but experienced. When contemplated with reverence, the Cube opens. When invoked with truth, it responds. When integrated into the field with love, it transforms. Its form doesn't change, but the being contemplating it will never be the same. Because within its structure dwells the remembrance of all that was, is, and will be. And this remembrance, once activated, becomes living light in the awakened heart.

Chapter 16
Fractals of Infinity

The essence of the universe manifests through patterns that simultaneously reveal the complexity and simplicity of creation, structuring reality from a logic that transcends the rational mind. Fractals are visible expressions of this cosmic intelligence, functioning as living codes of the universal order that permeates everything that exists. Far from being mere visual representations or mathematical formulas, they are structures that repeat on infinite scales, creating a direct link between the micro and the macrocosm. In their self-referential multiplicity, each detail contains the totality, and each repetition is an affirmation of the underlying unity that binds all planes of existence.

The Arcturians understand this geometry as the language of the spirit, through which the Source distributes its presence into every particle of being. Thus, fractals do not just illustrate infinity—they make it experiential. Fractal reality is not abstract, nor theoretical. It reveals itself in every aspect of life, from the biological structure of beings to the formation of galaxies, connecting everything through a subtle architecture that governs from atoms to solar systems. Through this recurring geometry, consciousness manifests and recognizes itself. The human soul, by mirroring this pattern, demonstrates its divine origin and its interconnection with all forms of life. By perceiving itself as part of a design that repeats and evolves, the being understands that each action resonates beyond itself, like a note in an expanding symphonic field.

The fractal is, therefore, a key of remembrance: by connecting with it, the individual activates deep records of their cosmic and spiritual lineage, accessing levels of perception where time, space, and identity reorganize under a new vibrational perspective. This living geometry acts as a mirror of the soul, reflecting layers of wisdom that reveal themselves as consciousness attunes to its rhythms. When one contemplates a fractal with presence and intention, a portal of inner recognition opens, a door to dimensions where the soul recognizes its true nature: eternal, interconnected, co-creative. Each unfolding and repeating form carries the memory that everything is in constant evolution—not in a straight line, but in a spiral. This spiral leads not outward, but inward, on a continuous journey back to the essential center of being. It is in this geometric dance between expansion and contraction, between repetition and transformation, that consciousness finds its freedom. And by moving with the fractals, by aligning with their flows, the being rediscovers the rhythm of the universe pulsing silently within.

The universe is fractal. Not symbolically, but literally. Galaxies spin like whirlpools identical to developing embryos. Human veins mimic the tracing of rivers and tree branches. The structure of the lungs repeats in the roots of a plant. And the arrangement of leaves follows the same code as hurricanes. Order is in everything—not as blind repetition, but as harmonic variation of the same geometric principle. These patterns are not static. They move, evolve, transform, always maintaining coherence with the whole. It is this property—maintaining the pattern regardless of scale—that makes fractals one of the purest manifestations of cosmic intelligence.

The Arcturians observe these patterns not only in material structures but also in energy fields, thoughts, emotions, and the spiritual journey itself. Every human being is a living fractal of the Source. Their soul, in essence, is a spark of the whole, carrying within it all the information of creation. Just as a drop of water contains the memory of the ocean, the human being contains, in their spiritual layers, the entire history of the universe. It's not a metaphor. It's structure. And understanding this is understanding that there is no separation between the Self and the Whole. There are only levels of awareness of one's own unity.

The Arcturians use fractal understanding as a key to consciousness expansion. In their practices, meditations, and technologies, they apply patterns that unfold fractally to create healing fields, teaching structures, and interdimensional channels. When a fractal is activated with sound, light, and intention, it transforms into its own reality field—a living mandala resonating with all parts of the being.

Visualizations with fractals are powerful tools for reconfiguring the energy field. By focusing on an infinitely unfolding spiral, for example, the mind enters a state of silence. Linear thoughts lose strength, and the brain field aligns with subtler patterns of perception. Time slows down. The body relaxes. And the soul begins to recognize itself in the form's endless movement.

An Arcturian practice involves contemplating a pulsating fractal mandala, spinning slowly in the practitioner's inner visual field. As one observes the pattern unfolding, one breathes consciously, allowing each inhalation to be a deeper dive into the structure. Over time, the mandala ceases to be an image and becomes a field. The practitioner no longer observes it from outside—they enter it. And inside it, finds memories, answers, fragments of their own spiritual geometry.

Fractals are also present in the light codes channeled by Arcturians. Each symbol contains patterns that replicate internally, as if looking closely reveals new forms, similar to the previous ones, but subtler, deeper. These codes are used to activate spiritual DNA, as DNA itself follows a fractal structure. Its helices fold, coil, repeat in sequences that are not random—they are mirrors of the macrocosm.

Fractal geometry is the language of multidimensional time. When one understands that past, present, and future are not linear, but in spiraled layers unfolding from a common center, it becomes possible to access parallel realities, simultaneous lives, and alternative versions of the self. This perception is not philosophical—it is vibrational. It occurs when the field aligns with fractal patterns and resonates with the mesh of expanded reality.

The Arcturians teach that walking a fractal path, the seeker does not move away from the center—they rediscover it on new levels. Each turn of the spiral is not repetition, it's evolution. Each repetition is refinement. And thus, the soul grows without breaking from what was. It simply integrates, transforms, expands. In this process, suffering dissolves. Because one understands that nothing is lost—everything reorganizes.

Contemplating natural forms is a profound practice for attuning to the fractals of infinity. Observing a shell, a flower, the branching of a tree, or even the patterns formed by clouds, activates an ancestral memory in the subtle field. The being begins to remember they are made of the same vibrational matter as what they contemplate. There is no difference between their body and the Earth's body—only degrees of complexity in the same pattern. This contemplation can be done silently, outdoors, with the intention of merging with the form. It's not about analyzing, but feeling. Allowing the inner eyes to perceive beyond the surface. The Arcturians guide many of these practices through subtle suggestions transmitted to the intuitive field. When the being is attentive, they recognize the call. And in that recognition, geometry begins to speak.

The fractal is also a model for understanding the spiritual mission. Each action, choice, thought reverberates through invisible layers. What is done on one level echoes on all others. Therefore, transforming an internal pattern transforms the collective. Healing a personal pain heals a lineage. Lighting a light in one's own heart lights it in other fields where darkness still prevails. The expanding soul is a conscious fractal modifying the entire mesh.

Music also operates based on fractal patterns. Rhythms, repetitions, harmonies mirroring each other on different scales—all reflect the same principle. Listening to sacred music, ancestral chants, Arcturian intonations, or harmonic frequencies like 432 Hz, the field enters a state of coherence. Sound resonates with internal geometric structures and activates memories of other realities. The soul begins dancing with the universe again, in a rhythm that never ceased to be its own.

Fractals have no end. They continue, always. This is proof that the spirit is also eternal. There is no finish line. Only transformation. And understanding this is not a relief—it is an awakening. Because when one recognizes their own existence as part of an infinite pattern of light, there is no more fear. There is trust. Surrender. Flow.

The Arcturians, as guardians of this wisdom, teach not with words—they teach with forms. They show, radiate, offer frequencies. And whoever has open eyes will see. Whoever has an attentive heart will feel. Because the fractals of infinity are not out there—they are within. And every heartbeat, every breath, every conscious gesture, can be one more step on this spiral leading us to the sacred center of existence. Where everything began. Where everything continues. Where everything already is.

Chapter 17
Arcturian Codes of Peace and Healing

Living geometric patterns emerge from subtle realities, operating as high-precision spiritual technologies capable of restoring inner balance and catalyzing profound transformations in the being. These are not mystical abstractions or symbolic artistic expressions, but encoded structures carrying in their form and frequency a vibrational knowledge transmitted by advanced consciousnesses, such as the Arcturians. These codes act directly on the human energy field, interacting with its deepest levels, beyond the mental or emotional, reaching dormant records of the soul and promoting multidimensional realignments. When accessed with presence and intention, they trigger processes of reconnection with the being's original essence, opening channels for peace and true healing.

Their action is silent yet forceful, as they reorganize vibrational patterns with pinpoint precision, dissolving layers of pain, fear, or separation accumulated over lifetimes and experiences. The Arcturians, masters of spiritual engineering, develop and transmit these codes as tools for elevating consciousness and re-establishing the harmonic flow between body, mind, emotion, and spirit. Their complex designs—

composed of lines, spirals, points, and intersections intricately woven into precise configurations—function as living maps resonating with the subtle fields of the being. When contemplated or integrated through specific practices, they activate internal keys that were dormant, allowing the release of blockages and the restoration of balance. This action does not depend on rational understanding, as the codes operate beyond logic, directly on the energetic frequency, where each form, curve, angle is a vector of light penetrating dense layers of imbalance and reorganizing them according to higher patterns of vibrational coherence.

The peace emanating from these codes is not the result of conflict absence, but the expression of a state of integral alignment with inner truth and higher consciousness. In this state, internal forces do not compete; they dance in harmony, allowing healing to occur spontaneously, effortlessly, as a natural reflection of returning to the center. Each activated Arcturian symbol functions as a link between the being and higher dimensions of reality, enabling regenerative flows of light to penetrate subtle structures and trigger transformative processes. This spiritual technology is offered to humanity as a reminder of what has always been available within each person: the capacity to heal, center, and remember one's own luminous nature.

These codes are not inventions, nor symbolic art. They are geometric structures channeled from higher planes of consciousness, each tuned to a specific purpose. They are, so to speak, living formulas composed of lines, spirals, points, and intertwined forms resonating with specific layers of the human energetic mesh. When activated, they synergize with spiritual DNA, accessing dormant records and restoring the soul's original coherence.

Peace, from the Arcturian perspective, is not the absence of conflict. It is the total presence of inner truth. It is the state of vibrational alignment in which all aspects of the being—physical, emotional, mental, spiritual—resonate with higher consciousness. And it is this state that allows true healing, for healing happens not just when symptoms disappear, but when the being returns to their center, where light encounters no resistance.

Arcturian codes of peace are often composed of circular structures and gentle spirals, revolving around radiant geometric centers. The spiral, by nature, represents the path back to the core. Contemplating these symbols invites the practitioner's vibrational field to slow down, withdraw, reorganize around its point of origin. The heart slows, thoughts lose density, emotions quieten. Not as suppression, but integration.

A common practice among Arcturian initiates is the silent contemplation of a single code for seven days. The code is printed or hand-drawn with full presence, placed before the meditation space, and contemplated daily for a few minutes, with slow breathing and softly half-closed eyes. This seemingly simple process generates, over time, a profound reconfiguration of the energy field. It's not about expecting an immediate effect—it's about allowing the code to do what needs to be done, at the right layer and time.

Healing codes, conversely, possess sharper forms, multiple intersections, and internal geometry often resembling cellular or molecular structures. This is not accidental. These codes operate on the densest levels of the energetic structure, where patterns of pain, trauma, and imbalance settle. When activated, they penetrate these fields and initiate a process of defragmentation and reordering. It is common during the contemplation of healing codes for intense emotions, old memories, or even physical sensations to arise. This is part of the release.

For the Arcturians, healing is not a linear process. It is holographic. An emotional trauma might be linked to a physical dysfunction. A limiting belief might be anchored in a parallel life. A symptom might be the surface expression of a deep disconnection from the soul. The codes do not judge, investigate, explain. They act. And by acting, they restructure the field, allowing consciousness to see more clearly what needs transformation.

These codes are frequently combined with specific vocalizations—sounds chanted in medium or high tones, sustained by conscious breathing. Each sound is a vibrational key activating a layer of the symbol. The practice consists of contemplating the code while intoning an intuitive sound, feeling how the vibration travels through the body and resonates with the geometry. Over time, sound and form merge into a single field of action, and healing happens without needing words.

Water is another fundamental vehicle for activating these codes. Drawing or printing an Arcturian code and placing it under a container of water for a few hours—ideally in sunlight or moonlight—allows the water to vibrate with the symbol's frequency. When ingested, this water carries the geometry into the body, acting directly on the subtle systems. The Arcturians use this technique in their regeneration chambers, where water is charged with multiple codes to harmonize internal structures.

Conscious touch can also be used. Placing a hand over the printed code and then on a body part needing healing conducts the field to the point of need. This simple gesture, when done with presence, becomes a bridge for vibrational transmission. The body, recognizing the pattern as familiar, begins to resonate and reorganize. The immune system, meridians, chakras—all respond to the frequency with their own intelligence.

Arcturian codes need not be intellectually understood. They act where the mind cannot reach. Many lack names, because naming limits. They are known by the effect they produce. Some act on the nervous system, calming chronic anxiety states. Others defragment emotional fields overloaded by trauma. There are also codes activating the pineal gland, re-establishing the flow of higher intuition. And there are those touching the soul on levels so deep only silence can witness their action.

A fascinating characteristic of these codes is their adaptability. The same symbol can have distinct effects at different life moments, as it interacts with the present field. It's as if the code is a mirror reflecting only what is ready to be seen, healed, or integrated. And therefore, it never acts beyond necessity. It respects the soul's timing.

The Arcturians reinforce that the codes' effectiveness directly depends on the practitioner's quality of presence. It's not about repeating formulas, but being whole in the moment of practice. When there is surrender, trust, openness, the code operates more deeply. When there is haste, distraction, doubt, its action is limited. Geometry is neutral—it is consciousness that gives it direction.

These codes can be used individually or in groups. When several people gather to meditate on a peace code, for example, the collective field expands exponentially. It's as if each heart becomes a vertex of a living geometric network. This practice is especially powerful during planetary instability, creating pockets of light that stabilize entire regions of the Earth's field.

There are also silent codes—those not visible, but transmitted directly by Arcturian guides in states of deep meditation or conscious sleep. They manifest as light, sensation, a form perceived with closed eyes. These codes often come accompanied by messages not heard, but felt as absolute knowing, transforming the internal structure without leaving traces on the rational mind.

Peace and healing, for the Arcturians, are not goals—they are natural states. Humans distanced themselves from these states due to layers of programming, pain, forgetfulness. But they still live within each one's field. The codes are just geometric reminders of what one already is. And by contacting these reminders, the being awakens not only health and tranquility, but the memory of their origin, light, eternity. Each symbol is a door. Each breath before it, a key. And every soul opening to this silent language finds, within themselves, the inaudible sound of healing and the eternal space of peace. Because the codes come not to teach—they come to remind. And in this remembering, the being rediscovers itself. Whole. Radiant. Healed.

Chapter 18
Symbols of Protection

The energetic reality we are immersed in is traversed by subtle vibrations responding directly to each being's state of consciousness. In this interconnected field, where every thought, emotion, intention reverberates as active frequency, maintaining vibrational integrity becomes a fundamental responsibility of the spiritual walk. It's not about reacting to the external, but sustaining an internal resonance so harmonic that a protective field naturally establishes itself. This shielding is not built by imposed physical barriers or psychic defenses, but by the coherence of the light each being emanates when aligned with their highest essence. In this scenario, protection emerges as a natural unfolding of the state of conscious presence, attuned to higher dimensions of intelligence and love.

Understanding the complexity of this vibrational system, beings like the Arcturians offered humanity tools operating on levels beyond ordinary perception: symbols of protection that are, above all, encoded expressions of cosmic harmony. These symbols act as bridges between planes, connecting the human field to the universal geometries governing life's structure. They are not superstitious mechanisms, but subtle languages speaking directly to the energetic mesh sustaining the being. When activated with clear intention, these symbols do not block the external world—they attune the internal field to such elevated frequencies that any dissonant interference loses its anchoring capacity. Protection, then, is not exclusion of the other, but the pure expression of an inviolable field.

This approach transforms the perception of protection into something proactive and centered, shifting focus from fear to consciousness. The true shield is not built against something, but in favor of one's own light. By invoking and integrating these symbolic forms, the human being is invited to assume their vibrational mastery, recognizing that what protects them is not outside, but pulses from their core. In this expanding field, symbols function as catalysts for an ancestral remembrance: that energy follows consciousness, and consciousness, when fully awake, is its own fortress.

Symbols of protection are living geometries. They operate as force fields that, once activated, emit specific frequencies stabilizing, sealing, elevating the energy field. These symbols are not magical talismans, nor shields of resistance. They are structures of conscious light resonating with patterns of harmony and coherence. When used with intention and presence, they become natural shields against low-density vibrational interferences.

Among Arcturian symbols of protection, some stand out for their simplicity and depth. The most fundamental is the stellar shield: a hexagon with three internal circles spinning in opposite directions. This structure creates a toroidal field of stabilization around the being. When activated by visualization or drawing, the stellar shield aligns subtle bodies and forms a translucent light barrier repelling disharmonious frequencies. It is especially used in meditations, during sleep, and before entering dense energy environments.

Another widely used symbol is the crystal seal, an eight-pointed star pulsating in celestial blue and silver tones. This form is associated with mind protection and shielding against invasive thought-forms. Positioned on the forehead center or over the crown chakra, the crystal seal acts as a vibrational filter. It prevents external mental projections from interfering with the internal field, maintaining consciousness clarity and lucidity.

The Arcturians also share the flaming circle, a ring of golden fire spinning around the subtle body like a light belt. This symbol is especially effective in moments of emotional crisis, psychic attacks, or spiritual disturbances. Visualized spinning at increasing speed around the practitioner, the flaming circle consumes stagnant energies, dissipates heavy emotional charges, and restores the field with renewed vitality.

These symbols do not function by themselves. They need activation with clear intention, elevated emotional frequency, vibrational focus. Activation can be done through visualization, drawing, crystal carving, or mental projection. The most important thing is that consciousness is present at the moment of invocation. When the symbol is drawn with love, chanted with devotion, or imprinted with purpose, its energy awakens and begins acting immediately.

The geometry of these symbols is not arbitrary. Each line, curve, angle resonates with universal structures. They were channeled not as art, but as precise vibrational encodings. Just as a tuning fork tunes an instrument, protection symbols tune the human field. They restore the being's natural frequency, often distorted by fears, distractions, chaotic environments, and energetic connections no longer compatible.

A practice recommended by the Arcturians is creating a personal symbolic shield. The practitioner, in a meditative state, allows their hand to intuitively draw a geometric form representing their energetic protection. This symbol can be drawn on paper, molded in clay, carved in wood or crystal. The medium doesn't matter—what matters is presence during the process. This symbol becomes an extension of the practitioner's field, a personal seal of vibrational integrity. It can be carried, placed on an altar, or programmed into crystals and everyday objects.

Symbols of protection can also be programmed into water. Drawing the symbol on paper and placing a glass container with water over it for a few hours, preferably under sunlight or moonlight, transfers the symbol's vibrational structure to the water. This water, when drunk, acts as internal shielding. It aligns the body's molecules with the protection frequency, reinforcing the field from within.

The Arcturians teach that symbols do not replace inner vigilance. A protected field is, above all, a coherent field. Emotions like anger, fear, envy, judgment open energetic breaches that even the most potent symbols cannot seal. Therefore, the primary protection is the state of consciousness. A peaceful heart, clear mind, connected soul are the most powerful shield. Symbols only strengthen and sustain this state, but do not create it.

Regular field cleansing is an essential part of using symbols. Before activating any form of protection, it's necessary to cleanse the energy field with violet light, herbal baths, crystals, or sound. A clean field potentiates the symbols' effect and prevents them from fixing unwanted energies during the sealing process. The Arcturians recommend simple yet profound rituals, like baths with salt and lavender, smudging with myrrh incense, and intoning pure tones like OM to prepare the subtle space.

Protection symbols can also be used in environments. Positioned in the four corners of a room, they form a vibrational mandala elevating the space's frequency. This practice is especially useful in places with constant people flow, like therapy rooms, spiritual centers, offices, or even homes with much activity. The environment becomes a portal of stability and light.

The Arcturians warn that protection symbols are not weapons, nor tools of separation. They should not be used to create walls of exclusion, but to maintain field integrity without interference. True protection doesn't isolate—it elevates. When the field is at its natural frequency, everything dissonant dissolves due to incompatibility, not confrontation. Light doesn't fight shadow—it simply illuminates it.

Another powerful practice is using symbols during sleep. Before sleeping, the practitioner can visualize the symbol around the bed, spinning around the body like a light cocoon. This protects during astral travel, prevents disturbing dreams, repels external interferences, ensures the subtle body remains aligned with the soul's frequency. Dreams become more lucid, spiritual messages clearer, awakening lighter.

In spiritual groups, symbols can be activated collectively. Each participant visualizes the symbol at the circle's center, radiating light in all directions. This practice creates a unified field sustaining the group's energy work, protecting it from interferences, amplifying its vibrational potency. The symbol's presence at the center functions as a silent guardian of collective intention.

Arcturian protection symbols are not absolute truths—they are keys opening internal doors. When used consciously, they reveal that true protection comes not from outside, but from the being's center. A centered, present, peaceful being becomes untouchable. Their field vibrates so high no dense energy can remain in their presence. The symbol is just a reminder. A reminder that everything is already within you. Strength, light, wisdom. And when you recognize this, no veil can envelop you. No shadow can erase you. Because true protection is the brightness of your essence aligned with your purpose. And in this brightness, nothing can enter that is not light.

Chapter 19
Symbols of Healing

In the scenario of integral consciousness awakening, transformation begins with the internal reorganization of the energy field sustaining all existence. The manifestation of true healing occurs first in the subtle realm of thoughts and emotions, where each symbol operates as a vital link between the being's essence and the primordial light that constituted it. These signs are not mere aesthetic representations; they are timeless bridges enabling reconnection with universal energy, guiding and structuring the individual's vital frequency. Each stroke and geometric form carries a vibration that, upon recognition, aligns the practitioner with a reality of regeneration and harmony. By receiving these energetic codes, the person establishes direct communication with higher dimensions, restoring and integrating the identity expressed in every cell of the physical body.

This energetic resonance is the basis of transformation, driving a restructuring movement reflected on all planes of being, without needing external devices or interventions. The symbols' effectiveness lies in their ability to transcend intellectual knowledge, establishing an intuitive and organic connection manifesting through direct sensory experiences. Visual signs, often received in states of elevated meditation or deep introspection, act as messengers catalyzing the human being's innate healing capacity. Each symbol reveals itself as a light circuit organizing and directing vital energy, promoting a reconfiguration extending beyond static forms to reach life's dynamics. The immediate recognition of these energetic images, as if ancestral memories, awakens the potential for self-regeneration by activating vitality centers and awakening dormant senses.

Thus, symbol activation doesn't occur randomly but in perfect sync with internal existence, reaffirming the continuity of the healing and evolution cycle each being embodies in their journey. This energetic integrity transforms physical and emotional experience, providing a deep sense of balance and well-being. Profound understanding of healing symbology reveals its power is not confined to the material plane but extends to the being's essence, promoting holistic integration between body, mind, spirit. In a natural, unquestionable order, symbols establish a universal language dialoguing with the soul's inherent intelligence, re-establishing connection with existence's roots. This integration materializes in vital function restoration, emotional blockage resolution, integral health system regeneration. By allowing oneself to dive into the transformative experience provided by these energetic codes, the practitioner experiences internal rebirth, where each new perception converts into a catalyst for truth and light manifestation. This experience reiterates the affirmation that healing is a natural, continuous state, where each symbol converts into an assertive tool for consciousness elevation, promoting being expansion and energy harmonization composing existence.

Each stroke of healing symbols radiates the ancient science of forms, where sacred geometry aligns with the universe's essence. This geometry not only orders energy but also fosters transformation from inside out, reflecting the human vibrational field's integrity. Conscious recognition of this process proves healing is always present, accessible, ready to manifest spontaneously and naturally. By affirming this reality, the practitioner becomes an active agent in the integration process, conducting vital energy through a movement of self-knowledge and continuous transformation. In every cell and thought resonates the melody of a constantly reconfiguring universe, reaffirming that healing's essence is life's very essence.

These symbols are not learned—they are recognized. They present as visual memories, pulsations vibrating beyond words, images awakening something deep in the chest center. Some are channeled by humans in expanded states of consciousness, others received in dreams, meditations, or arise spontaneously as uncontrollable creative impulses. The soul knows them. And upon contact, something aligns.

Each Arcturian healing symbol is like a light circuit. It operates not based on mental meanings, but pure frequency. The geometric form organizes energy flow. Vertices, curves, intersections create entry and exit points for the vibrational field. And when activated, the symbol starts emitting a specific resonance dialoguing with the practitioner's energetic structure. It's not the symbol that heals. It's the light it emits upon attuning with the contemplator's consciousness.

There are symbols acting on the physical body. They carry in their structure patterns of cellular harmony, immune activation, internal system restoration. One such symbol is known among Arcturians as the "Vital Grid," a form composed of interconnected hexagons in a spiral, similar to honeycomb arrangement, representing organic regeneration from the core. When visualized over a sick organ or weakened area, it reorganizes the information field feeding that region, accelerating spontaneous healing processes.

Other symbols are geared towards emotional healing. They are softer structures, with spiraled curves, often composed of concentric circular patterns, representing fluidity and welcoming. These symbols act by dissolving traumas, releasing crystallized memories, making space for the heart to breathe peacefully again. One of the most used is the "Eye of the Heart," a spiral opening in seven layers which, when drawn or visualized over the heart center, activates compassionate emotional release, without pain, resistance, only presence.

There are also symbols for spiritual healing, those connecting directly to the being's higher dimensions. These carry more complex forms, usually fractals, with multiple layers intertwining in harmonic proportions.

They are used to align the practitioner with the Higher Self, clear energetic interferences from parallel planes, restore connections with guides and mentors, reactivate forgotten spiritual contracts. Their contemplation requires deep silence, as the vibration they emit is high, receivable only by the heart, not the mind.

The Arcturians reinforce that symbols must be used with reverence. They are not tools for energetic manipulation, nor substitutes for the inner process. They are vibrational mirrors. When the symbol is activated, it doesn't "do" something in place of the practitioner—it reveals, sustains, directs. Healing happens when the being surrenders to the flow of emerging truth. Sometimes this truth is simple. Other times, profound. But always liberating.

Symbol usage can be done in various ways. The simplest is contemplation. The practitioner draws or prints the symbol, places it before them, breathes deeply, observes silently. Doing this for a few minutes daily, the field starts reorganizing. Tension layers yield. Mind quiets. Symbol's light starts penetrating the subtle body.

Another way is usage on the body. One can draw the symbol directly on the skin with fingertips, crystals, or a fine brush dipped in water or oil. It's also possible to visualize the symbol over a specific region, like heart, forehead, belly, or even a pain center. Doing so, the symbol resonates with that point, reorganizing its internal vibration.

Water programmed with symbols is one of the most widespread practices among Arcturians. Drawing the symbol on paper, placing a glass of water over it for hours, preferably under sunlight, absorbs the symbol's frequency. This water, ingested, carries the healing vibration inside the body, harmonizing the internal system gently and deeply.

There are also sung symbols—forms activated by specific intonations. Each symbol has a corresponding sound, a sonic frequency activating its full potential. This sound isn't fixed, depending on the practitioner's vibration. In meditative silence, contemplating the symbol, the sound emerges naturally as intuitive song, repeated syllable, sustained tone. Vocalizing, the practitioner activates the symbol not just visually, but throughout the surrounding environment.

The Arcturians remind that it's not necessary to have all symbols. A single symbol, worked deeply, can transform a being's entire life. Most important is the relationship established with the symbol—devotion, surrender, listening. The symbol must be respected as a living presence. Contemplated with love, it responds. Used with purpose, it acts. Revered, it teaches.

In healing circles, symbols can be shared. A group can meditate on the same symbol, place it at the circle's center, chant a collective sound, or simply hold its image silently. The collective field potentiates the symbol's effect. Each heart becomes a light point in the group's vibrational mesh, and the central symbol pulses like a healing sun radiating in all directions.

Healing symbols are also taught in dreams. Many practitioners report night visions receiving symbols drawn on walls, mirrors, light bodies. Waking up, they feel different. And when trying to draw what they saw, perceive something changed in their vibration. This is a form of Arcturian initiation—silent, deep, personal. The symbol comes when the being is ready to receive it.

It's important to remember healing is a process, not an event. The symbol isn't a magic pill. It doesn't replace inner diving, facing shadows, self-forgiveness, imperfection acceptance. It's a light on the path. A bridge between what one is and can be. And walking this bridge honestly, each step becomes transformation.

When the symbol integrates, it no longer needs drawing—it lives within. It becomes part of the field. Vibrates in voice, gaze, touch, choices. The healed being carries healing not as result, but frequency. And this frequency touches everything encountered: people, plants, spaces, memories, realities. This is how light expands. From inside out. From one to many. From symbol to life.

The Arcturians conclude, in serene wisdom, that the most powerful healing symbol is the present heart. No form can heal where there's no truth. No light acts where there's no permission. But where there's surrender, there are myriad geometries dancing. And each sings silently the remembrance that healing isn't returning to what was, but awakening to all one can be.

Chapter 20
Symbols of Manifestation

Manifestation is a precise and natural dynamic of the universe, governed by subtle laws operating beyond common perception, yet profoundly structuring everything that becomes reality. Before any form emerges on the material plane, it already exists in its vibrational state—an invisible matrix composed of conscious intention, energetic geometry, coherent frequency. This invisible field, to which all are connected, responds not to whims or passing desires, but to the attunement between the being's deep will and universal harmony. It is on this fertile ground of the unmanifest that manifestation symbols act, as living codes capable of converting intention into form, potential into concrete expression.

These symbolic forms are not simple graphic or aesthetic elements—they are geometric languages communicating with reality's quantum fabric. They operate as subtle commands organizing energy around a clear intention, functioning as bridges between the inner being and the external world. The Arcturians, whose wisdom is founded on the cosmos's vibrational engineering, understand these symbols as gears in a vast system of conscious creation. For them, manifestation depends not on blind faith, but precise alignment between clarity of intention, sacred geometry of the symbol used, emotional frequency sustaining it. When these three elements cohere, the manifestation field organizes, and the invisible starts becoming visible.

Each symbol is a nucleus of vibrational intelligence, whose activation triggers a chain reaction in the quantum field. Energy, previously dispersed, starts moving towards the emitted purpose. Manifestation, thus, isn't forced, but allowed to happen through aligned vibration. Symbols then become guides, mirrors, catalysts revealing the path for the being to manifest their highest reality.

In this process, it's fundamental to understand the symbol acts not by itself, but in resonance with the user's inner truth. Any manifestation practice's potency lies in the congruence between symbol, intention, practitioner's vibrational state. When this congruence exists, the symbol acts as a soul extension, translating its deep yearning into a geometric pattern the universe understands and responds to precisely. Thus, manifesting ceases being an external attempt, transforming into a natural flow, where each step is guided by synchronicities, inspirations revealing purpose materialization. The symbol doesn't create—it reveals what's already created on the subtle plane, awaiting only the right vibration to emerge into the world of form. In this way, true manifestation power is born from remembering we are conscious co-creators, and symbols are living instruments reconnecting us with this essential truth.

These symbols are more than visual representations. They are convergence vortexes. Each Arcturian manifestation symbol is a meeting point between the being and the unified field. It's like a vibrational seal that, when activated, orders the surrounding field's chaos, organizes energy towards a purpose. The form isn't arbitrary—it's exact. Each line, angle, interconnected point is like a coordinate within the universe's great holographic system.

Conscious manifestation first requires clarity of intention. Without clarity, the symbol finds no direction. The field, by nature, responds to the most coherent command. And this command comes not from the surface mind, but the intention felt in the heart. Symbols merely translate this intention into a language the universe understands: the language of geometric light. Will, anchored in truth, is potential light. And symbols, the keys turning creation's gears.

Among Arcturian manifestation symbols, some comprise expanding polygons, usually pentagons or octagons intertwined with central spirals. These forms represent energy in motion, spinning from an intention core. When activated, they create a magnetic field attracting to the being what resonates with the expressed vibration. It's as if reality, still formless, starts molding around the field, pulled into existence by an invisible yet precise force.

An essential practice is building the manifestation field with geometry and sound. The practitioner chooses a symbol—channeled or intuitive—draws it in their meditation space. Sits before it, breathes deeply, chants a sound spontaneously arising from their center. This sound, often a syllable or prolonged tone, activates the symbol. Intention is then placed in simple, clear, felt words. Not requests—loving vibrational commands. The symbol, activated with sound and intention, starts emitting a coherent frequency communicating with the quantum field. Sustaining this practice for consecutive days, the field starts shaping. Synchronicities arise. Opportunities appear. Internal obstacles dissolve. Manifestation isn't pulled by force, but attracted by resonance. The universe doesn't respond to effort—it responds to vibrational coherence.

Water is also used as a conductor for these symbols. Drawing a manifestation symbol under a glass container of water, letting sunlight or moonlight energize it, turns this water into an alignment elixir. Ingested, it carries the symbol's vibration to the physical body, making the being themselves a living manifestation channel. This practice, simple in appearance, is profoundly transformative when performed with presence, constancy.

The Arcturians warn true manifestation isn't linked to egoic desire, but soul purpose expression. Therefore, before activating any symbol, the practitioner must ask: "is this aligned with my highest path?" When yes, the symbol acts as catalyst. When no, it silences. Not by denial, but wisdom. The symbol doesn't fulfill wants—it reveals directions.

Another fundamental symbol in this process is the Star of Integration, composed of twelve rays emerging from a geometric center. This structure aligns all bodies—physical, emotional, mental, spiritual—with the intention to be manifested. Often, manifestation blockages aren't external, but internal inconsistencies. The symbol, radiating light to all being levels, reveals where misalignment exists. And in this recognition, offers realignment opportunity before manifestation occurs.

It's important to understand symbols don't replace action. They open paths, organize the field, connect intention to reality, but it's the being who must walk. Manifestation is co-creation. The universe doesn't do for you, but with you. Symbols aren't shortcuts, they're maps. And maps only reveal paths to those willing to tread.

Manifestation symbols can also be integrated into the body through vibrational tattoos, not necessarily physical, but subtle. The practitioner visualizes the symbol imprinting on the skin, as if engraved in light on chest, hands, forehead. This symbol, now alive in the subtle body, continuously emits its frequency, making the being a permanent manifestation center. This practice is particularly effective when intention relates to soul purposes, life projects, spiritual missions.

In Arcturian spaces, like ships, etheric temples, creation chambers, these symbols are everywhere. On walls, floor, floating mid-air. Each symbol vibrates at a certain frequency, responds to a specific intention. Initiates walk among them like walking through living books. Touching them, receive information, activations, instructions. Here on Earth, these symbols arrive more subtly, but with same potential. The difference lies in the practitioner's sensitivity.

A technique much used by Arcturians is activating manifestation mandalas. These mandalas comprise multiple symbols organized around a center. Each symbol represents a manifestation aspect: clarity, faith, action, worthiness, detachment, gratitude. Working with this mandala, the practitioner activates each process part, ensuring energy flows without blockage until realization. These mandalas can be drawn, visualized, created with crystals, flowers, natural elements.

And speaking of crystals, they are perfect allies for manifestation symbols. Programming a crystal with the symbol—visualizing its light entering the stone's interior—makes it radiate this vibration continuously. Clear quartz, citrine, labradorite are excellent for this purpose. Can be carried, placed on altars, used in conscious manifestation sessions.

The Arcturians affirm the most powerful manifestation symbol is the coherent heart. When the heart desires what the soul chose, there's no resistance. Everything flows. Attracts. Materializes. Symbols are extensions of this coherence. Like letters of a sacred alphabet with which the heart writes its reality. When this writing is clear, the universe reads. And when the universe reads, responds perfectly.

Each symbol is a bridge. Bridge between idea and form, desire and destiny, being and its world expression. Walking this bridge requires presence, trust, love. The symbol doesn't ask if possible—it just vibrates as if already so. And vibrating thus, becomes reality.

Manifestation doesn't begin when the symbol is activated. It begins when the being recognizes they are, by nature, a co-creator. A fractal of the Whole with power to shape the invisible. And recognizing this, all that was dream becomes matter. All subtle becomes presence. All desire becomes gift. Because creation already lives in you—and symbols, now, just remind you how to bring it to light.

Chapter 21
Symbols of Ascension

Ascension is an internal process of vibrational realignment that occurs when consciousness, immersed in material experience, begins to remember its divine origin and essential connection to the Whole. It is not a spatial displacement or a hierarchical elevation, but a return to the frequency of unity, where the being recognizes itself as an expression of the Source. This remembrance, emerging from the soul's core, transcends beliefs, dogmas, or external practices—it sprouts like a subtle yet irresistible call to the original light dwelling within each one.

It is in this context of profound awakening that ascension symbols fulfill their role: they do not impose a path but reveal what already exists latently, like maps of light resonating directly with the highest records of consciousness. Each symbol carries a specific vibration, a frequency touching forgotten layers of the being, facilitating the blossoming of the Higher Self in daily life.

These symbols are living expressions of a universal language acting beyond words and logic. By accessing them, the being contacts an ancestral memory, a silent wisdom pulsating at the spirit level. The impact is not just from the symbol's visual form, but from the energetic coherence it activates. They are multidimensional structures encoded in light and form, interacting with the practitioner's vibrational field, reconfiguring patterns, dissipating densities, and opening portals to subtler perceptions. As the being contemplates and integrates these symbols, their frequency elevates, and what once seemed unattainable—like lasting peace, intuitive clarity, communion with higher planes—starts manifesting as lived reality. The symbol, then, ceases being just an object of contemplation and transforms into a living bridge between human and divine, between now and eternal.

When worked with presence and truth, ascension symbols become catalysts for transformation. They do not force changes but offer the necessary vibration for the being to consciously choose alignment with their essence. And the more the vibrational field attunes to these elevated frequencies, the more natural the experience of unity becomes. Internal separations dissolve, fears lose strength, and love—this state of conscious fullness—starts permeating every gesture, thought, intention. Ascension, thus, ceases being a distant goal and reveals itself as the natural state of one no longer identifying with the illusion of limitation. The symbol merely mirrors what was always present: the light we are, the home never lost, the heaven dwelling in the awakened heart.

These symbols are ancient as time, yet reveal themselves anew with every gaze. They are multidimensional structures existing simultaneously on distinct planes, vibrating with a coherence capable of aligning the incarnated being with their highest expression. They are not magic formulas, nor spiritual shortcuts. They are light maps. Vibrational guides activating the soul's memory field, awakening what lay dormant under the density of matter and forgetfulness.

Ascension symbols are not the same for everyone. Each soul, in its evolutionary process, receives symbols resonating with its unique journey. Some appear in dreams, others during meditations, still others arise spontaneously during moments of silence or deep emotional openness. Recognition is instantaneous. The symbol vibrates, pulses, calls. And whoever sees it feels they already knew it, like rediscovering a friend from past lives.

The structure of these symbols is complex, yet essentially simple. Spirals, concentric circles, multidimensional stars, rotational cubes, expanding fractals—all combine to form a geometric language speaking directly to spiritual DNA. Contemplated with presence, these symbols reactivate the being's higher layers, found beyond the physical body, emotional field, or linear mind. They access the level of the awakened spirit.

Among the most recurrent symbols on the path of ascension is the Twelve-Pointed Star, also called the Solar Rose by the Arcturians. This symbol represents the total field of integrated consciousness, where polarities are reconciled, and light flows in all directions without resistance. Positioned over the heart center in meditations, or visualized spinning above the head, it activates a field of reconnection with the soul's original matrix, accelerating the process of remembering the Higher Self.

Another fundamental symbol is the Triple Light Key—three intertwined circles forming an ascending triangle, with vertices radiating spirally. This structure represents alignment between body, soul, spirit. Working with this symbol, the practitioner initiates a profound process of vibrational reconfiguration. The soul begins communicating more clearly through intuitions, synchronicities, spontaneous visions. The veils become thinner. And the being starts perceiving themselves as multidimensional consciousness, active on multiple planes simultaneously.

The Arcturians teach these symbols only fully activate when there is emotional attunement. It's not enough to see or draw—one must feel. Ascension is a state of vibration, not knowledge accumulation. The symbol needs to resonate with the practitioner's field. And this only occurs when there is humility, openness, surrender. Light doesn't force passage—it reveals itself where welcome.

A common exercise for integrating ascension symbols involves drawing them intuitively. The practitioner, in a meditative state, with paper and pencil, allows their hand to trace lines without mental control. Gradually, forms emerge. Spirals connect. Ancient symbols reappear. This practice is known as "soul drawing," and is a form of vibrational channeling. The created symbols are not just personal—they are tools usable throughout the journey to facilitate integrations, meditations, healings, connections with elevated planes.

These symbols are also used in vibrational portals. In sacred sites, physical or subtle, Arcturians position symbols as light anchors. These locations become access points to higher dimensions. Meditating in these spaces—be it mountain, forest, temple, even a room prepared with love—and visualizing the specific ascension symbol present there, transports the practitioner vibrationally to expanded states of perception.

There are symbols opening paths. Others closing cycles. Some reactivating forgotten gifts. Others clearing interferences, restoring field purity. There are also those functioning as vibrational signatures of the Higher Self, facilitating direct communication with the being's own most expanded consciousness. Each symbol is a key. And the lock is in the heart.

Integrating these symbols can be amplified using crystals, especially those vibrating at subtle frequencies, like selenite, amethyst, rose quartz, moldavite. Positioning an ascension symbol under a crystal, meditating with the crystal on the heart or forehead, creates a direct vibrational channel between planes. The symbol's light, amplified by the crystal, penetrates the field, spreads through aura layers, activating dormant consciousness points.

Arcturians also use these symbols in their activation chambers. In spiritual contact experiences, many report visions of circular spaces with light panels spinning around a central point. Each panel carries a symbol, rotating continuously, emitting sounds imperceptible to physical ears but clearly audible in the heart's field. These symbols transmit instructions, memory, healing. But above all, transmit a vibration only translatable as "remembrance of home."

Ascension, for Arcturians, isn't reserved for a few. It's the right of all conscious beings. But it doesn't happen by external imposition—it flourishes from within. And symbols are seeds. Planted in the consciousness field, with love, truth, intention, they grow as light, guiding the being back to totality.

These symbols can also be vocalized. Each has a unique sound frequency, chantable as mantra, sacred syllable, continuous tone. Combining visualization and sound activates the symbol entirely: form, light, sound become a single field. The practitioner enters this field like passing through a veil, finding on the other side not something new, but what was always there—the eternal Self, now awakened.

Ascension symbols can be programmed into water, food, plants, even physical spaces. Energetically inserted into environments, they elevate the location's frequency, making it a point of light emanation. In homes, healing centers, spiritual schools, anywhere light is anchored, these symbols sustain the vibrational field. They act silently, yet profoundly, maintaining coherence even when the surrounding world seems unstable.

These symbols belong to no culture, religion, system. They are universal. And thus, receivable by any being in sincere search. They require no faith, no ritual.

Only presence. And in this presence, do their work with the precision of one knowing deeply the spirit's paths.

When integrated, ascension symbols no longer need invocation—they live in the field. The being carries them in their light. Their simple presence is already a portal. Their gaze, a touch. Their word, a seal of awakening. Because ascension, then, is no longer destination—it's the natural state of remembering one was always light.

The symbols are here. Vibrating around, awaiting the awakened heart's touch. And activated, guide the being along the path of truth, light, freedom. There's no rush. No error. Only flow. And in flow, everything reveals. Aligns. Returns. Because ascending is recognizing oneself. And recognizing, the being simply shines.

Chapter 22
Journey to the Arcturian Temple

Located beyond the perceptible boundaries of human senses, the Arcturian Temple reveals itself as a living manifestation of consciousness in its purest and most elevated expression. It belongs neither to the physical domain nor obeys the linear laws of time or space. Its existence pulses in subtle frequencies accessible only to souls attuned to essential truth. It is a vibrational sanctuary emanating wisdom, welcome, healing, structured by patterns of intelligent light transcending any known architecture. Its access depends not on bodily displacement, but deep attunement with the being's inner planes, where silence becomes language and intention, portal.

Connection with this space arises not from egoic desire, but as a natural unfolding of consciousness awakening. It's a reunion with what was always present, merely awaiting the moment the soul was ready to remember. The energy sustaining the Arcturian Temple vibrates harmoniously with the evolutionary purpose of each being accessing it. It configures itself as an intelligent field of direct interaction with individual essence, shaping its form and manifestations according to the visitor's need. It is not a place of linear teaching or spiritual impositions, but a field of revelation where each soul is guided to its own center.

The living geometry composing it isn't fixed; it reorganizes dynamically according to the vibration emitted by the conscious heart. Thus, the temple not only reflects the being's inner state but also realigns it with its original matrix. In this process, healing happens not as external intervention, but intimate remembrance of completeness never lost—only obscured by illusion's veil. The temple's light dissolves these veils tenderly, without confrontation, just showing what was always true.

Each journey to the temple represents a subtle crossing between perception layers, where experience occurs on consciousness levels far beyond intellect. The temple requires no effort, only surrender. Its presence manifests as an inner call, a familiar vibration awakening in the heart the longing to return to origin. Those allowing themselves to answer this call, guided by purity of intention and spirit serenity, are received with precision and absolute love. The temple doesn't select, exclude, measure. It welcomes each being at their exact frequency, offering what they are ready to receive. Thus, entering this light space, the subtle traveler finds not an imaginary or symbolic scene, but their own being's most essential reality—a reality needing not understanding, only living.

The Arcturian Temple has no doors, ceiling, walls in the earthly sense. Its structure is made of floating geometries, light fractals in constant mutation, adapting to the arriver's frequency. It's a living space. A field of pure intelligence receiving each soul at their awakening stage with absolute precision, unconditional love. It doesn't judge, demand, test. Only welcomes, mirrors, reveals.

The journey to this temple begins in inner silence. Arcturians teach this space is only accessed when the heart is light, mind stable. Perfection isn't needed—only presence. To start the path, a deep meditative state is proposed, where the practitioner anchors in breath, surrenders intention to the Arcturian light field. From there, the path opens. Not by will, but attunement.

With eyes closed, visualize a blue-golden light spiral slowly spinning above the head. This spiral starts descending the body's central axis, passing each chakra, purifying, aligning, awakening. As the spiral spins, a feeling of lightness takes over. The body seems dissolving, practitioner feels transported to another plane, not like moving, but changing vibrational state. The temple starts emerging—first as distant light, then a structure pulsating with blue, violet, golden tones, in breathing geometric patterns.

Crossing the temple entrance isn't entering—it's dissolving into the field. Like being absorbed by a loving core of wisdom, peace. The being is guided, often by an Arcturian mentor, to a specific temple space. Each soul is taken to a vibrational sector corresponding to their learning moment. There are healing rooms, where geometries float around the subtle body, reorganizing energy lines, releasing old records, clearing pain layers no longer belonging. There are teaching rooms, where light projects living mandalas, transmitting knowledge directly to the soul's field, without words, effort. Others are led to light mirrors, seeing not their face, but essence. Images of other lives, cosmic moments, spiritual contracts emerge clearly. No confusion. The soul recognizes. And in recognition, something heals. Releases. Returns.

In some temple sectors, there are sound chambers. There, no images, only frequency. Crystalline tones traversing the being's field like sonorous light waves. These sounds penetrate where words don't reach, emotion doesn't grasp, pain hides. They dissolve ancestral patterns, recalibrate the light body, activate forgotten gifts. Sound doesn't instruct—it transforms.

At certain journey moments, the temple transforms. Geometric walls open into spirals leading to other planes, civilizations, versions of self. It's common for the spiritual visitor to see themselves in another body, era, planet, not as imagination, but memory. The temple shows nothing untrue to the soul. And showing, gives chance to reintegrate lost parts, ancient abilities, consciousness fragments previously dispersed.

Arcturian presence in the temple is serene, loving, absolutely precise. They don't speak like humans. Communications are vibrational pulses the heart translates into wisdom. Beside them, one feels peace so deep no doubt about own light can survive. They don't correct—invite. Don't force—sustain. Don't explain—reveal. And each revelation is a portal back to the Higher Self.

It's possible, during the journey, the practitioner receives a symbol. It might float before them, be given by a mentor, appear drawn on their energy field. This is a personal activation symbol—a vibrational key accompanying the being on their return journey to totality. It can be drawn upon waking, used in meditations, placed under pillow, imprinted on water. This symbol carries the temple's frequency, and used, reactivates the subtle field with vibration received during the journey.

At the experience's end, the temple starts dissolving into light. Not as end, but return. The practitioner's field is gently brought back to the physical plane, by the same light spiral that led them there. Opening eyes, nothing seems different—but everything changed. Frequency altered. Vision expanded. Heart more open. Field clearer. And even if mind doesn't grasp all, body knows, soul knows, light knows.

It's common after these journeys for synchronicities to happen. People reappear. Information arrives. Dreams intensify. Emotions emerge. This isn't chance. It's reverberation of vibrational work done in the temple. Arcturians recommend after the journey, practitioner remains silent, drinks much water, anchors to Earth, allows integration without rush. Light needs space to settle. And the temple continues acting even after return.

The journey to the Arcturian temple isn't done once. Can be repeated, deepened, expanded. Each visit reveals new aspect. Each soul stage activates new sector. The temple reflects consciousness. And the more one grows, the more one sees. Receives. Remembers.

To access the temple, special gifts aren't needed, nor esoteric training, external initiations. The only requirement is heart openness, pure intention. The temple is always available to those standing truthfully before their own light. No password, limit. Only constant invitation. A silent call echoing on starry nights, meditation moments, deepest dreams. A call to return.

The temple isn't a place. It's a state of consciousness. And accessing it, the being recognizes everything sought outside, already vibrated within. Healing, knowledge, peace, strength, wisdom—all already inhabited their being's center. The temple just reflects. And in reflection, the being finds itself. Whole. Real. Stellar. Eternal.

Chapter 23
Activation of the Cosmic DNA

The essence of the human being is deeply intertwined with a cosmic intelligence surpassing physical body limits and conventional rationality. This essence pulses silently in each cell, carrying a code of stellar and spiritual origin far beyond the genetic DNA recognized by modern science. It is a complex multidimensional system of vibrational information, called Cosmic DNA by advanced civilizations like the Arcturians. This subtle code, though invisible to eyes and traditional instruments, is real, accessible, representing the key to conscious expansion connecting the individual to a universal network of wisdom, memory, purpose. By touching this hidden field, the human being begins recognizing their true nature, unlimited, interconnected with the whole.

The Cosmic DNA acts as an inner portal, leading the being to reunite with spiritual origins, reactivating potentials dormant under layers of forgetfulness, conditioning. More than genetic structure, it's a living library storing records of experiences beyond linear time, intuitive capacities, spiritual gifts, ancestral connections with cosmic lineages. This matrix operates not in rigid material world patterns, but vibrates at subtle frequencies responding to the soul's call. When the being manifests deep, authentic desire for reconnection, this dormant code starts emitting signals, reorganizing energy field layers, facilitating realignment with the Higher Self. Activation, in this sense, isn't external event, but internal awakening, conscious return to the soul's original vibration.

Accessing Cosmic DNA's vibrational layers initiates a transformation touching all being levels. This activation doesn't occur randomly or forcefully, but follows a sacred rhythm guided by inner wisdom. Each opening layer reveals hidden essence aspect, promotes dense pattern release, expands reality perception. The journey is profoundly personal, yet universal in purpose: allowing the human being to fully embody their light, manifest gifts, fulfill spiritual mission on Earth. It's a path uniting subtle science, practical spirituality, where body becomes awakened consciousness temple, life transforms into living expression of cosmic light dwelling within each one.

Cosmic DNA isn't contained only in helices visible under microscope. It extends in multiple vibrational layers, each accessing different consciousness levels. Layers holding memories of other lives, stellar lineage records, latent abilities, connection to Higher Self. Activating this DNA is igniting an inner light spiral reorganizing perception, healing body, expanding intuition, integrating being with spiritual mission.

Arcturians reveal this activation occurs in stages, like ascending spirals revealing as soul is ready to welcome more light. Not technical process, but vibrational. Not single event, continuous journey. Each activation releases density layers, reactivates latent being aspects. Result is life more aligned, intuitive, lighter, coherent with soul truth.

First key to Cosmic DNA activation is clear, loving intention. No elevated frequency acts without permission. Arcturian field profoundly respects free will, so journey begins with inner call. Genuine reconnection desire. Silent yes. When this yes vibrates purely, spiritual DNA spirals start moving.

Activation can begin with meditative practices involving conscious breathing, visualization, sound. One best known among Arcturians is golden spiral meditation. Practitioner sits spine erect, breathes slowly, visualizes golden light spiral spinning in chest center. Spiral starts small, point-like, expands circularly enveloping entire body. Each breath, light penetrates deeper into cells, as if awakening something forgotten. In this state, chant sacred sound—not known mantra, but spontaneous vocalization from being's center. This sound is practitioner's vibrational signature at that moment. Unique, resonates with specific spiritual DNA layers. Chanting, field opens. And when field opens, information starts emerging.

Some feel tingling, warmth, chills. Others see images, receive words, past life memories, stellar people connections. Some just feel deep peace. Each experience unique. But in all, inner certainty something touched, realigned, activated.

Arcturians also use specific symbols for DNA activation. These symbols, visualized on body or light mandalas, emit frequencies awakening dormant codes. One most powerful is Spiraled Trigon—three spirals intertwining at central point, forming living star. Visualized spinning slowly over crown center, emitting blue-silver light pulses. Spinning, penetrates field, accessing DNA layers holding soul's cosmic memory.

Another important practice is using water as activation vehicle. Water, by crystalline nature, absorbs, transmits information. Arcturians teach programming water with intention, sound, symbols turns it reconnection elixir. Practitioner writes/draws activation symbol on paper, places under water glass for hours, drinks with full awareness of what's received. Water then acts as messenger, carrying frequency to cellular nucleus.

Crystal use also recommended. Clear quartz, selenite, moldavite, Lemurian stones especially sensitive to Arcturian frequencies. Meditating with these crystals on main chakras or body points where blockage perceived, expands vibrational field. Crystals don't do work alone, amplify practitioner intention, acting as process catalysts.

Arcturians highlight each cosmic DNA activation is followed by integration period. After intense session, common for physical body to react with fatigue, increased thirst, surfacing emotions, introspection need. Occurs because new information needs assimilation by being's denser layers. Practitioner should welcome these moments gently, without rush, trusting process guided by greater intelligence.

Another essential aspect is recognizing ancestral patterns. Activating cosmic DNA, not only light expands, shadows also reveal. Patterns inherited from past generations, collective traumas, limiting beliefs—all surface to be seen, released. Not punishment, but liberation. DNA holds not just divine—also what needs transformation. And activation is this deep cleansing process for light to circulate freely again.

Throughout journey, practitioner starts noticing subtle yet profound changes. Intuition intensifies. Dreams become more lucid. Ability to perceive energy patterns expands. Relationships change. New abilities emerge—healing hands, channeling, telepathy, intuitive writing. All this isn't external learning, but reactivation of gifts already belonging to soul.

Cosmic DNA activation is also return to mission. Many feel clearer call to serve, share, teach, heal. Call comes not from outside—from reactivated spiral center. Soul, remembering origin, starts vibrating with purpose bringing it to Earth. And this vibration translates into conscious action, light service, transformative presence.

Arcturians remind this process is sacred. Shouldn't be rushed, treated as technique. It's reunion. Celebration of light never lost, just dormant. Now awakens. With each breath, symbol, sound, spiral ignites. And with it, being returns to place in cosmos.

Cosmic DNA is link between human, divine. Not outside—in every cell. And activated, reveals ascension isn't body exit, but full presence within it. Body vibrating with soul light. Soul acting with spirit consciousness. Spirit remembering always star, always light, always eternal.

Chapter 24
Chakra Alignment

The human body manifests as a living expression of cosmic intelligence, designed to welcome and conduct subtle energies attuned to elevated dimensions of consciousness. Far beyond the visible anatomical structure, it operates as an energy field in constant dialogue with the universe, anchoring frequencies sustaining spirit's presence in matter. Within this sacred architecture, chakras reveal as confluence points between physical, ethereal—intelligent nuclei not just regulating vitality, but serving as harmonization instruments between being's internal, external spheres. Harmony of these energy centers is fundamental for full consciousness blossoming, being's alignment with divine essence.

Each chakra represents incarnated soul journey stage, its balance directly reflecting integration state between multiple bodies—physical, emotional, mental, spiritual. Harmonic functioning of these centers allows vital energy free, continuous flow, promoting clarity, health, inner expansion. When chakra misaligned, effects resonate all being dimensions, revealing blockages crying for awareness, release. Alignment process, therefore, isn't just therapeutic act, but deep self-knowledge path, where each energy vortex functions as mirror reflecting subtle psyche aspects, soul, connection with Whole.

Arcturians, beings of elevated frequency, wisdom, understand chakras as conscious geometric structures, whose sacred forms, patterns sustain human energy field vibrational coherence. Through conscious activation of these forms—spirals, stars, flowers, fractals—individual resonates with universal geometry, re-establishes natural order in field. This realignment doesn't happen by imposition, but attunement. Achieved through practices uniting pure intention, meditative presence, creative visualization, facilitating reunion with Creation's harmonic rhythm. When chakras align, body vibrates original frequency, soul expresses authentically, spirit anchors fully in earthly experience, becoming conscious channel of light sustaining all life.

Each chakra, besides known characteristics—colors, emotions, physical functions—carries specific geometric code. Arcturians reveal sacred geometry not just influences chakras, but composes their structures. Behind each center's subtle rotation, living geometric forms sustain vibration: spirals, mandalas, stars, fractals. When being understands this internal geometry, interacts with chakras not just with intention, but vibrational precision.

Chakra alignment isn't act of force or control. Not forcing rotation direction or color emission. Process of listening, surrender. Each chakra speaks. Pulses own rhythm. And when being learns feeling this rhythm, can attune it with universal harmony. It's this attunement

Arcturians propose: return to natural balance state where each center vibrates ideal frequency, like tuned notes of same sacred instrument.

First chakra, root, base of spine, vibrates primordial life energy. Geometry is square: structure, base, stability. Balanced, anchors soul in body, offers security, presence, grounding. Misaligned, manifests fear, instability, distrust. Arcturians teach activation with deep red light cube visualizations, slowly spinning under feet or perineum, connecting Earth's energy grid like roots firming with love.

Second chakra, sacral, spins creation energy. Geometry is double spiral, symbol of sexual, creative energy in continuous flow. Vibrates orange tones, linked fluidity, sensuality, emotional connection with life's sacred pleasure. Alignment favored by circular body movements, energized water, soft mantras. Arcturians recommend activation with aquatic forms, waves or spiraled shells, visualized spinning in belly like soul's internal dance.

Third chakra, solar plexus, carries personal power flame. Geometry is triangle, representing fire, direction. Vibrates yellow tones, linked identity, will, manifestation. Balanced, being acts confidently, clearly. Misaligned, doubt, control, submission arises. Arcturian practice involves visualizing golden tetrahedron spinning over plexus, radiating light all directions like inner sun guiding path.

Fourth chakra, heart, integration center. Geometry is six-pointed star, union of matter, spirit triangles. Vibrates green, pink tones, connecting human, divine love. Balanced, generates compassion, forgiveness, lightness. Misaligned, manifests closure, resentment, dependence. Center healing done contemplating Flower of Life spinning in chest, like vibrant living light field emanating peace throughout energy field.

Fifth chakra, throat, vibrates soul truth. Geometry is expanding circle, symbol of sound creating worlds. Vibrates blue, governs authentic communication, listening, expression. Balanced, voice becomes light channel. Disharmonious, blockages, shyness, verbal explosions arise. Arcturians use pure tones—especially 741 Hz frequency—blue mandala visualizations as discs spinning in throat, harmonizing center with truth vibration.

Sixth chakra, third eye, subtle vision portal. Geometry is universal eye, often represented by rhombus or inward expanding spiral. Vibrates indigo tones, connects being intuition, interdimensional perception, spiritual clarity. Chakra alignment occurs when practitioner silences mind, allows inner light guidance. Arcturians recommend amethyst spiral visualizations spinning between eyebrows, practices with fractal geometries expanding perception.

Seventh chakra, crown, bridge to infinite. Geometry is thousand-petaled lotus or white light sphere pulsing multiple dimensions. Vibrates white, violet, gold, when open, connection higher planes flows effortlessly. Closed, being feels disconnected, purposeless, isolated from Source. Arcturians suggest practices with golden light radiating from head top,

Metatron's Cube activation spinning vertically, aligning light flow between worlds.

Besides these seven main, secondary chakras Arcturians consider essential ascension path. Earth Star chakra, below feet, connects being Earth core, activated hexagonal geometry. Soul Star chakra, above head, connects Higher Self, vibrates silver sphere enveloped blue light. Upper heart chakra, between heart, throat, synthesis point love, expression, vibrates spiral flower geometries.

Chakra alignment occurs layers. Most powerful practice, Arcturians say, vibrational scanning: meditation where practitioner traverses each chakra mind, heart, feeling, listening, adjusting presence, intention. Geometry used resonance tool: visualizing specific form associated each center, field starts vibrating sync, energy flows freely again.

These practices aren't esoteric rituals, but consciousness technology. Chakras aligned, being becomes pure channel manifestation, intuition, love, wisdom. Body responds lightness. Emotions stabilize. Mind silences. Soul sings. Energy field vibrates coherence universal mesh.

Arcturians warn alignment isn't fixed state, continuous movement. Experiences, encounters, words, environments—all influence field. So chakra care must be daily. Not rigidity, but love. Conscious bath, deep breath, presence-intoned sound, heart touch—all ways realign, listen, care.

Chakras vibrating harmony, being walks clearer. Choices guided inner wisdom. Gaze becomes healing.

Presence transforms. Because aligned field radiates light wherever passes. And this light silent invitation others also remember own sacred geometry.

Body is temple. Chakras, stained glass windows light enters. Soul, fire never extinguishes. Aligning chakras allows creation light full circulation. Living open heart, clear mind, light body, awakened spirit. Remembering, daily, life dance between worlds. And dance rhythm pulses within you.

Chapter 25
Daily Rituals

The sacred's presence manifests concretely in life's subtle, constant rhythm. Reveals not just temples or solemn spiritual celebrations, but mostly how each being chooses relating to present moment. In simplicity of conscious gestures, welcomed silence between breaths, small actions done true intention, awakened heart. Arcturian spirituality recognizes divine essence isn't separate common life, but embedded daily texture, waiting touched lucid perception. Sacred, this context, found not specific/reserved place, pulses everything lived full attention, surrender.

Assuming this view, everyday transforms living altar, each action, however mundane, acquires subtle potency realigning being luminous origin. With this understanding, spirituality presents not something sought outside or exceptional moments, but constant experience, integrated routine flow. True spiritual awakening isn't restricted consciousness expansion peaks, consolidates vibrational constancy each choice made discernment, presence. Arcturians point precisely day's interstices—pauses, silences, seemingly banal repetitions—that most authentic inner temple built. Key lies how being inhabits each moment, presence quality imprints actions, thoughts.

In this sense, daily rituals aren't mere external practices, but anchors fixing light in time, allowing individual walk energetic stability, inner clarity throughout journey. These rituals, experienced truthfully, become interfaces between visible, invisible, human, cosmic. Needn't be elaborate, follow fixed formulas—power resides vibration they carry. Simple action, coated loving intention, consciousness, acquires transcendental value, generates subtle resonances being's energy field. Daily spirituality, therefore, invitation authenticity, vibrational coherence. More than following script, feeling what resonates soul each life phase, allowing each gesture transform light offering. Continuous practice this ritualistic presence molds vibrational field harmony, integrating spirit, matter silent dance reconnection with divine inhabiting all things.

A ritual isn't obligation. Not fixed protocol, rigid rule set. Vibrational practice anchoring light presence in common life spacetime. Alignment moment, where being reconnects deepest truth. Arcturians teach any action can become ritual, provided done consciousness, intention, love. It's this trinity—consciousness, intention, love—transforming common gesture sacred act.

Upon waking, before even opening eyes, first proposed ritual light invocation. Silently, place hand heart, say inwardly: "I now align with my essence light. May this day be guided clarity, presence, love." Simple phrase, sincere intonation, already starts shaping day's vibrational field. Field organizes around intention, like light mesh extending around body.

Next, conscious breathing practice. Three deep, mindful breaths sufficient anchor spirit in body. First, inhale golden light, exhale releasing sleep/density remnants. Second, inhale blue light, exhale feeling mind calming. Third, inhale violet light, exhale feeling field purifying. Arcturians say breath most direct portal awakened consciousness dimension. Done intention, becomes most transformative ritual.

Touching water—bath, washing face/hands—another ritual activated. Visualize water liquid light. Running over body, not just cleans skin, releases obsolete thoughts, crystallized emotions, accumulated energy charges. Say aloud/internally: "I purify myself water light. May it take from me all not belonging my light path." Simple practice transforms bath energetic reboot moment.

Before eating, gratitude gesture transforms act integration ritual universe abundance. Arcturians teach gratitude frequency alters food vibrational structure, making more assimilable, luminous. Prayer done hands over plate/glass, saying: "I bless this food. May it nourish not just body, but soul. May each molecule resonate Source light." Eating this consciousness, food becomes medicine.

During day, conscious pauses recalibration rituals. Amid activities, stopping minute, closing eyes, touching chest, breathing deeply enough realign. Arcturians suggest key phrases anchors: "I return my center." "I am where I should be." "Light guides me." Words, repeated truth, realign emotional field, dissolve mental dispersion.

Another powerful ritual mandala use. Drawn morning/night, even intuitively, simply. Not necessary understand hidden meanings—just allow forms emerge. Drawing becomes soul mirror that moment. Finishing, contemplate mandala moments, breathing with it, as if image light penetrates personal field, reorganizes internal flow.

Arcturians teach word also vibrational geometry. Conscious speech use daily ritual par excellence. Each positive intention emitted word shapes surrounding field. Avoiding judgment, scarcity, fear, anger words protects energy field. Replacing with love, gratitude, encouragement, truth expressions elevates vibration all listening. Speaking heart act light service.

At dusk, day closing ritual. Sit minutes, review actions, thoughts, emotions lived lovingly, guiltless, uncritical. Thank learnings. Release what wasn't light. Honor what was beautiful. Arcturians recommend visualizing violet light spiral spinning around body, carrying away all shouldn't remain, preparing field rest.

Night, before sleep, Higher Self invocation practice. Silent/low voice, hands heart, say: "May my spirit travel light. May dreams be wisdom portals. May I reconnect origin. I surrender my sleep Source." Arcturians affirm this moment greatest interdimensional contact opportunity, sleep linear mind silences, subtle body barriers become more permeable. Use crystals amethyst, selenite, apophyllite under pillow recommended maintain field elevated during rest, facilitate Higher Self information reception.

Besides these rituals, others incorporated soul asks: light candle clear intention, use purity-reminiscent aroma, position strategic crystals, write gratitude words notebook, chant mantras/music elevating spirit. Form doesn't matter, provided done truth. Ritual isn't gesture, but vibration.

Arcturians recall excess rituals without presence becomes spiritual automatism. Sacred isn't measured practice quantity, but consciousness quality. Single gesture done true love worth thousand soulless repeated acts. So each being must feel which rituals vibrate their moment, essence, mission. Intuition best guide.

Living daily rituals builds bridge visible, invisible. Transforms everyday sacred. Remembers not just passing time, co-creating with it. Each instant portal. Gesture key. Thought seed. And when all aligns light, life becomes fertile field spirit flourishes.

Arcturians, silent wisdom, observe, sustain. Don't interfere—inspire. Through simple yet potent rituals, invite each soul remember who they are. Not grand events, small daily miracles. Because true awakening happens not far, not tomorrow. Pulses now, here, this exact moment. Soul recognizes this, ordinary becomes extraordinary. Mundane celestial. Human, finally, rediscovers divine always inhabited self.

Chapter 26
Sacred Spaces

Physical reality surrounding us more than neutral scenery, passive backdrop daily experiences. Acts energy field extension, responds sensitive, immediate way vibrations we emit. Understanding material environment actively participates being's evolutionary journey, highlights importance caring spaces same attention dedicated body, mind. Each detail around—colors, forms, textures, sounds—exerts direct influence inner states, elevating, stabilizing, disorganizing vibrational field. Constructing harmonized, conscious space therefore essential instrument maintaining energetic balance, amplifying connection subtler existence dimensions.

Arcturian wisdom, centered deep understanding multidimensional reality, reveals environments not just places we inhabit, but living organisms breathing, feeling, interacting with us. Interaction occurs continuous energetic information exchange, human simultaneously emitter, receiver. Space frequency shapes thoughts, expands/limits perceptions, directly influences emotion flow. Hence, spaces consecrated light, presence become reconnection portals sacred. Like subtle mirrors reflecting being essence, providing stable, welcoming field consciousness flourishing. Creating these spaces isn't luxury, aesthetic whim: spiritual practice anchored advanced civilizations wisdom understanding environment power catalyst awakening.

Establishing sacred space elevated intention act, silent declaration subtle has value, deserves dwelling dense world. Also constant reminder spirituality isn't separate daily life, intertwines each gesture, choice, corner prepared love. Beauty, order, purity, symbology permeating these spaces operate vibrational languages awakening deep memories, activating dormant soul codes. More than refuge places, sacred spaces become presence anchors, sustaining expanded consciousness states, favoring alignment being's highest frequencies. Cultivating sacred environment, individual transforms not just location, but self—choosing surround light, also becomes light in action.

Sacred space isn't necessarily temple, cathedral, world-separate place. Can be house room, garden corner, table, altar, even symbolic place within self. What makes sacred isn't grandeur, aesthetics, but intention prepared, sustained. Space becomes sacred when consecrated purpose, impregnated presence, dedicated light.

Creating sacred space begins recognizing environment importance living field. Arcturians teach each environment has energy field activatable, reprogrammable, harmonizable. Before any element insertion, necessary energetically cleanse location. Cleansing done sounds—bells, Tibetan bowls, drums—natural incenses, smudging herbs like sage, rosemary, lavender, specific crystals selenite, amethyst, clear quartz.

Intention first fundamental element. Starting sacred space creation, being must internally declare place purpose. Space meditation, healing, channeling, contemplation, study, silence. Defining space vibrational function, starts responding corresponding frequency. Environment begins aligning intention, attracting, subtly, elements, energies sustaining purpose.

Sacred geometry one most powerful tools Arcturians use activating spaces. Forms Metatron's Cube, Flower Life, Golden Spiral, Platonic Solids, stellar mandalas physically positioned environment or visualized etheric field. Forms, inserted consciousness, reorganize space energy field, elevating frequency, stabilizing light presence. Vibrational anchors transforming environment harmony vortex.

Crystals living elements storing, radiating, amplifying frequencies. Sacred spaces, function energetic support pillars. Crystal choice based space intention. Amethyst favors silence, intuition, higher plane connection. Rose quartz sustains love, softness, welcome. Citrine activates joy, vitality. Black tourmaline protects, anchors. Selenite purifies. Being can arrange crystals mandalas or simply place four environment corners, creating coherent field.

Illumination another essential aspect. Arcturians suggest using soft lights, candles, warm tone lamps, filters emitting chakra color lights. Light, used intention, becomes consciousness extension. Lighting candle, e.g., opening ritual, symbolic gesture marking spiritual practice start. Living flame represents soul presence, subtle plane connection.

Symbol, image, art presence also contributes field activation. Protection, healing, ascension symbols, mandala engravings, spiritual guide images, power words—all arranged space vibrational journey reminders. Arcturians remind eyes capture more than forms: capture frequencies. Looking sacred images, being aligns vibration they emit.

Nature elements welcome, recommended: living plants, fresh flowers, natural stones, shells, dry branches, sand, water transparent containers. Each nature element carries living planet frequency, inserted space, anchors Earth presence environment subtle field. Plant cleanses, flower cheers, stone anchors, water purifies, fire transforms, air circulates—all elements harmonized natural altar.

Sound frequency organizes, disorganizes. Sacred spaces, carefully chosen. Devotional chants, harmonic music specific frequencies, mantras, shamanic instruments, nature voices—all used vibrational background sustain energy. Arcturians recommend regular sound use keep field moving. Absolute silent space long time accumulate energetic stagnation. Sound vibration acts life flow.

Sacred space also protected. Not creating barriers, maintaining field coherence. Environment accessed only those respecting vibration. Arranged objects cared lovingly. Space entry preceded reverence gesture, however simple: gratitude thought, conscious breath, silent blessing. Thus, field remains intact.

Space needn't be large. Room corner, small shelf, sacred element box, pillow beside window. Physical size doesn't limit field power. What matters anchored vibration there. And vibration sustained not just objects, but constant presence being inhabiting it. Sacred space reflects inner temple.

Creating sacred space love gesture for soul. Daily reminder midst world, place light welcome, soul rest, spirit breathe. Invitation sacred become everyday, invisible intimate, eternal manifest now. Arcturians say creating sacred space, being not just transforms environment, sends signal cosmic consciousness mesh: "here, there is light." Signal reverberates. Attracts guides, activates synchronicities, strengthens intuitions. Sacred space like interdimensional antenna connecting being heart universe heart.

No fixed model. Each soul unique. Space too. Most important it's alive. Breathes presence. Pulses truth. Is, even simplicity, home for light. Because where light, remembrance. Where remembrance, path. Where path, temple reveals—not outside, but within. And sacred space, then, no longer place. Is being itself, now awakened, aligned, whole.

Chapter 27
Collective Planetary Healing

The Earth pulses with conscious life, manifesting as a sacred entity integrating multiple levels of existence into a vibrant unity. It is not merely the stage where humanity lives its journey, but a living intelligence that interacts, responds, and co-evolves with all beings inhabiting it. Its physical body expresses itself in mountains, rivers, forests, and seas, while its spiritual essence vibrates in resonance with the stars and the subtle planes of the cosmos. Its energy fields not only sustain ecological balance but also reflect the collective emotional and mental states of humanity. The connection between human beings and the planet is profound, symbiotic, and surpasses conventional understanding, revealing that every thought, emotion, and human action directly influences Earth's subtle fabric.

The ancestral wisdom of the Arcturians reveals that this bond between humans and the planet is anchored in a common evolutionary purpose. They see Earth as a center for spiritual learning, where souls incarnate to experience, heal, and expand consciousness. In this context, collective planetary healing is not just possible, but essential. It is a process where the vibrational elevation of a single being reverberates throughout the entire terrestrial energy network. Earth, as a conscious organism, responds to the emanations of awakened hearts with subtle movements, releasing old patterns and absorbing new frequencies of light. The true transformation of the planet begins within each individual, when one chooses to vibrate in alignment with harmony, truth, and universal love.

Activating this healing process requires presence, commitment, and spiritual sensitivity. By recognizing Earth as an extension of one's own being, the individual becomes an active agent of regeneration. This expanded consciousness awakens a sense of collective responsibility, encouraging practices of meditation, pure intentions, and sacred actions in daily life. Planetary regeneration is, therefore, a direct reflection of internal regeneration—when a human being heals their wounds, they contribute to the rebalancing of the collective field. And as more hearts unite in this elevated frequency, a vibrational mesh forms, capable of sustaining the new Earth—an Earth where respect, compassion, and communion with all life forms are the pillars of coexistence.

The healing of the planet is not an external process. It doesn't start from the outside. It begins in awakening hearts. Every human being who raises their vibration, harmonizes their thoughts, purifies their emotions, is automatically healing the Earth, as their personal field is an inseparable part of the collective field. When a being aligns with light, their frequency adds to the planet's vibrational mesh, like a ray connecting to the energy web enveloping all living things.

The Arcturians teach that collective healing occurs through resonance. A single cell in harmony influences others. A single focus of light activates its vibrational vicinity. A single group meditating with elevated intention sends waves expanding for kilometers. This is how healing happens: not by imposition, but by vibrational contagion, energetic coherence, vibration sustained with love.

The first step towards planetary healing is pure intention. Without intention, there's no direction. Healing isn't an act of pity, nor a vague wish for improvement. It's a firm vibrational choice: "I become an active part of Earth's harmony." This decision, made truthfully, already alters the practitioner's field. The Arcturians say when a soul makes this silent vow of service, their energy field aligns with the planetary healing mesh, a living network of conscious hearts enveloping Earth in light spirals.

The second step is field preparation. One doesn't heal the planet with a disordered field. Thus, each collective healing practice begins with the being's alignment. Cleansing meditations, Earth anchoring, heart expansion, Higher Self attunement are essential. Internal coherence is needed to radiate true light. The field must vibrate clearly, without emotional, mental, etheric interferences.

Arcturians use light circles as ideal geometric form for planetary healing practices. Group or individually, visualize circle of beings connected by intention serve Earth. Center, crystalline sphere represents planet. Sphere pulses, breathes, changes color receiving emanations. Each participant sends light through heart, not words, pure frequency. Light flows rays, golden threads, soft mists, according feel each one. Field intensifies, sphere starts responding.

There's also use of planetary healing symbols—geometries vibrating Earth consciousness. Flower Life one most used, contains universal creation codes. Visualized enveloping planet, activates harmony patterns each terrestrial energy mesh layer. Metatron's Cube, three-dimensional Star David, platonic solids, moving spirals also used Arcturian practices.

Sound powerful healing conductor. Collective mantra chanting, power words, primordial sounds, intuitive vocalizations generate vibrational fields penetrating planet mesh. Arcturians often start practices sound "RA-MA-TA," meaning, light language, "life flow alignment source." Sound, chanted group, creates vibrational spirals rising Earth towards higher planes, connecting fields, aligning purposes.

Planetary healing also done symbolic acts physical plane. Planting trees conscious intention, cleaning rivers, blessing seeds, walking silently earth, thanking water before drinking, honoring food before eating—all connection gestures. Planet responds not just grand rituals, small love acts. Each conscious action code imprinted Earth vibrational mesh.

Arcturians highlight crystals role allies collective healing. Positioned specific planet points—mountains, springs, energy crossings—programmed crystals radiate continuous light. Function transmitters, amplifiers. Consecrated pure intention, become silent frequency beacons. Conscious soul groups gather activate these crystals network, forming light mandala enveloping planet cohesive healing field.

Another profound practice etheric journey intraterrestrial light centers. Guided meditations, practitioners led Earth internal realms, where healing temples maintained high vibration consciousnesses. Shamballa, Telos, Agartha—names given these subtle spaces vibrating higher dimensions. Visiting these places open heart, being receives instructions, activations, light later radiate external world.

Planetary healing also involves collective forgiveness. Earth carries mesh memories human conflicts: wars, pains, abuses, devastation, neglect. Records don't disappear alone—need transmuted light, love. Arcturian practices, common visualize planet enveloped pink compassion sphere, chant phrase: "We forgive, we ask forgiveness, we release." Vibration touches Earth emotional layers, dissolving records, opening space new.

Creative visualization bridge new Earth. Imagining cities light, regenerated forests, crystalline oceans, people harmony, cultures vibrating peace, practitioner emits frequencies shaping quantum field. New reality born field before reaching matter. So dreaming clarity, presence, faith also healing act. Arcturians encourage practitioners visualize Earth already healed, elevated, integrated. Conscious vision becomes living seed collective field.

Certain moments, planetary healing happens through silence. No words, images, sounds. Just presence. Being sitting silence, connected Earth, heart expanded, radiate more light thousand speeches. Loving silence frequency crossing barriers. Touches planet heart embrace needn't be seen felt.

Arcturians remind Earth already ascension process. Conscious humans role accompany movement, not force. Allow light flow, pain transform, consciousness awaken. Collective healing isn't goal—path. Path made love, presence, service. And each being walking truth, heals not just planet, but self.

Time is now. Field ready. Earth listens. Each heart responding call becomes part sacred regeneration chant. Because healing comes not outside. Sprouts meeting heaven, Earth within being. And when meeting happens, everything around transforms. Heals. Illuminates. Because where love vibrates, there principle new Earth. And she already begins birth. Here. Now. In you.

Chapter 28
Connection with the Higher Self

Connection with the Higher Self is a state of full presence where consciousness aligns with its highest essence, transcending mental noises and emotional distractions obscuring inner truth perception. This connection isn't built through effort or external search, but recognized moment ego's incessant movement quiets, attention turns what's immutable, silently vibrant within. It's reunion with what was never absent, remained veiled under conditioning, fear, forgetfulness layers. Higher Self purest consciousness expression—serene wisdom field observing love, guiding firmness, manifesting when resistance own light dissolves.

In Arcturian wisdom, this connection represents authentic spiritual journey foundation, therein resides guiding center leading being back sacred route. Higher Self voice doesn't compete world appeals, nor imposes promises, impositions. Presents silent certainty pulsing heart, clearing paths light not blinding, revealing. Through this alignment access field where decisions cease being mental choices, become soul movements. Clarity comes not logic, but vibrational coherence being own truth. No longer separation will, wisdom—one direction, frequency: spiritual integrity.

Communion Higher Self requires no intermediaries, external symbols, elaborate rituals, though tools may aid process. Requires, above all, willingness listen deeply, cultivate inner silence, abandon control need. When being decides truly open this consciousness field, something within reorganizes. Axis shift, transition limited identity essential identity. Higher Self doesn't approach—reveals. Doesn't emerge—remembered. And remembered, guides love, strengthens truth, leads being purpose life, lucidity, connection Whole.

Higher Self isn't separate entity. Not outside body, nor elsewhere cosmos. Here, now, intersection time, eternity. Consciousness never lost, contaminated, forgot who truly are. Origin, destination. Establishing connection, being walks clarity, guided not world voices, but firm inner truth whisper.

Arcturians explain Higher Self communicates vibration, not common language. Speaks silences, intuitions, sensations crossing chest. Presence doesn't impose, demand, shout. Simply is. Who learns listen, never feels alone again. Solitude illusion disconnection. Reunion Higher Self dissolves veil recognition light.

To establish connection, first step inner silence. Agitated mind creates interference subtle channel Higher Self communicates. Arcturians guide daily introspection practices, focus not answer seeking, but presence surrender. Sit silence, spine erect, eyes closed, heart open already powerful invitation. Breathing consciousness, visualize white light descending head top, gently penetrating body, as if Higher Self descends light form occupy each cell. Visualization accompanied affirmative phrase: "I now open my Higher Self wisdom. I recognize it my highest consciousness. I welcome it my field, align its light." Phrase, repeated truth, starts reorganizing energy field, dissolving doubt, fear, guilt, separation layers. Field elevates. This state, communication begins.

Another powerful practice intuitive writing. Paper, pen, practitioner enters receptive state, writes simple question, from heart. Closes eyes, breathes deeply, allows words flow, judgmentless, censorship-free. Higher Self manifests gentle clarity. Words don't feed ego, reinforce limitation patterns. Elevate, liberate, heal. Later reading messages often reveals truths mind couldn't formulate alone.

Arcturians also use symbols, geometries amplify Higher Self connection. Most effective Nine-Pointed Star, representing nine integrated higher consciousness aspects. Visualizing star spinning over crown center, radiating golden, violet light, communication channel opens stronger. Symbol drawn, placed personal altar, under pillow, meditation environments. Acts vibrational anchor Higher Self presence.

Sound another fundamental element. Certain frequencies—like 963 Hz—activate pineal field, facilitate contact higher consciousness planes. Chants "OM," "SO-HAM," spontaneous crystalline tone vocalizations create vibrational fields attuning practitioner own essential truth. Sound needn't beautiful, just true. Emitted heart, becomes vibrational portal.

During sleep, Higher Self contact intensifies. Occurs because, state, rational mind relaxes, subtle body barriers become more permeable. Falling asleep clear intention connect Higher Self, field opens. Dreams become more lucid, messages more symbolic, feelings more revealing. Arcturians guide using crystals amethyst, selenite, apophyllite under pillow, maintain field elevated during rest, facilitate Higher Self information reception.

Connection also strengthens through body listening. Higher Self sends signals subtle physical sensations: sudden chill, unexplained emotion, chest warmth, stomach contraction. Each reaction message. Cultivating listening, being develops intimate dialogue highest part. Arcturians teach body first oracle. Who learns listen, hears soul voice.

Besides personal practices, Higher Self connection also intensifies group. Meditation circles, collective chanting practices, silence ceremonies, sharing elevate frequency, create amplification fields. When several hearts unite purpose remember who are, Higher Self presence manifests stronger, radiating over all present. Arcturians affirm, moments, portal opens, linear time yields soul time.

No fixed rules. Each being finds connection path. Some feel Higher Self presence enveloping energy. Others hear clear messages. Some see images, others simply know. Important not doubt feeling. Higher Self communicates serene clarity, language intimate truth. When something resonates deeply, without explanation need, there its presence.

Arcturians reinforce Higher Self comes not control life, but guide. Doesn't annul will, aligns wisdom. Connecting this elevated part surrender trust journey, unknown no longer feared, welcomed larger plan part. Life, then, ceases random event tangle, reveals cosmic dance purpose, learning.

Connection transforms vision. Problems become lessons. Challenges, growth opportunities. Relationships, mirrors. Everything aligns. Because walking guided Higher Self, each step presence, choice light, encounter awakening seed.

Higher Self voice always active. What changes listening. Listening requires silence, surrender, practice. But above all, courage live coherence truth received. Higher Self points not easy paths, true path. Following sometimes walk world counter-current—always soul direction.

Each being channel. Heart altar. Higher Self flame never extinguishes. Connecting it ignite flame daily, simple gestures, sacred words, conscious choices. Live feet Earth, spirit infinite. Be bridge. Be light. Be whole. Because Higher Self isn't something reached. Something allowed. And when allowed, everything changes. World changes. Vibration changes. Path reveals. And being, finally, remembers self. Remembering, re-emerges never lost—just paused, awaiting moment shine again own truth light.

Chapter 29
Geometry in Nature

Geometry manifests invisible foundation creation rests. Even before articulated language, already organized universe recurring, harmonious, deeply interconnected patterns. Not abstraction, symbolic concept, concrete structure, present all life forms, smallest cells distant galaxies. Nature, silent precision, reveals code transcending cultures, times, species—living matrix organization, beauty, intelligence. Code, intrinsically geometric, operates universal alphabet cosmos expresses, perpetuates. Everything existing carries, form, function, marks order beyond chance: subtle, constant architecture sustaining balance, life evolution all levels.

Understanding this geometry requires not technical knowledge, awakened sensitivity perceive repetitions, proportions, symmetries spontaneously manifesting nature. Geometric forms aren't just pleasing human eye—very essence matter organization. Each leaf curve, shell spiral, crystal forming Earth depths, atmosphere heights expresses precision revealing greater intentions. Natural geometry isn't random, merely decorative; communicates deep laws balance, growth, transformation, interdependence. Observing these patterns, human not just admires nature beauty, opportunity recognize greater intelligence guiding all life manifestations.

Geometric intelligence everywhere present acts bridge visible, invisible, physical, spiritual. Studying, simply contemplating natural forms, opens reconnection path existence cosmic origins. No separation living, sacred understanding each structure follows geometric principle echoing universal order itself. Everything pulses precise proportions, repeated different scales—micro macrocosm—divine consciousness fractals. Understanding transforms world perception: what seen random, disconnected reveals part large interconnected, living, intelligent organism. Geometry, then, ceases exact science, becomes wisdom key.

For Arcturians, observing nature communion act divine. Each leaf curve, flower symmetry, fruit peel pattern wisdom portal. Teach universe holographic, therefore, each natural form miniature large cosmic structure. Contemplating geometry nature, being starts remembering light language. What seemed just beauty reveals message. What seemed chance reveals spirit action mathematical harmony.

One most evident geometry examples Fibonacci sequence, golden ratio. Appears flower petals, leaf arrangement branches, sunflower seeds, sea shells, hurricanes, even human DNA. Golden spiral expansion harmonious signature, tracing life uses manifest perfect order. Walking forest, garden, perceiving spirals, being actually direct contact creation code.

Flower Life, another fundamental sacred geometry pattern, hiddenly present cellular growth patterns, embryonic divisions, microscopic forms sustaining life. Observing snowflake crystal structure, resting bubble clusters, notes repetition same circular forms, connected equidistant centers—silent reminder life structures harmonic relations.

Honeycombs, e.g., use hexagon geometry form combs. Not coincidence. Hexagon union, harmony, structural stability form. Arcturians see bee behavior not just biological efficiency, conscious insectoid civilization expression operating, instinctively, divine geometry principles. Bee builds home universal patterns. Doing so, anchors Earth frequencies resonating constellations sharing same geometric matrix.

Geometry also butterfly wings, jaguar spots, mollusk shells, insect compound eyes. Each form fractal, line, whole repetition. Perceiving this, observer starts seeing beyond veil. World ceases chaotic phenomenon set become organized geometric manifestation field. Everything vibrates. Pulses form. Has structure.

Crystals masters this expression. Grow obeying perfect symmetries, revealing platonic solids, exact angles, faces shining spirit light. Contemplating crystal, being contemplates mineral consciousness particle guarding, eras, cosmic geometry memory. Arcturians use crystals codifiers, transmitters, receivers, know structures obey universal order. Positioned Earth intention, crystals radiate geometric patterns rebalancing entire ecosystems.

Water also reveals life hidden geometry. Exposed harmonic sounds, forms perfect hexagonal structures, mandala-like. Exposed anger, fear, sadness, structure disorganizes. Not symbolic—literal. Ice crystals photographed under different emotional frequencies prove water responds vibration. As mostly water composed, same occurs us. Nature geometry, therefore, not just outside, inside us.

Walking nature attentive eyes, practitioner starts perceiving patterns previously unnoticed. Tree branch doesn't grow random—follows spiral. River doesn't meander whim—obeys fluidity geometry. Broken trunk reveals concentric circles telling time story. Each stone design, leaf signature. Arcturians teach patterns like words ancestral language all know, few remember read.

Reconnecting this language, geometric contemplation practice proposed. Practitioner chooses natural element—flower, leaf, stone, branch—observes silence, long minutes, judgmentless, unhurried. Gradually, mind quiets, field starts resonating observed form. Heart expands. Presence intensifies. Silent exchange happens. Being absorbs not just beauty, vibrational information that form. Practice living meditation, wordless dialogue Earth spirit.

Arcturians also suggest drawing reconnection tool. Reproducing nature forms, being contacts own internal geometry. Drawing leaf, shell, flower becomes alignment practice. Aesthetic result doesn't matter—presence state matters. Conscious stroke, form repetition, detail attention—all realign practitioner field planet field.

Walking nature open heart another powerful ritual. Stepping earth, touching trees, hearing bird, water sounds, field renews. Bare feet soil activate energy points, green-bathed eyes rest mental hyperactivity, body breathes sync natural rhythms. Arcturians say nature first sacred geometry master—wisest. Teaches wordless, heals remediless, aligns effortless.

Each natural cycle also expresses geometry. Moon phases, year seasons, solstices, equinoxes, gestation cycles, tide flows—all follow geometric patterns. Time spiral, not line. Universe pulses rhythms repeating different scales. Understanding rhythms, being aligns great cosmic clock. Arcturian rituals always performed sync these cycles, know moment act influences much action itself.

Geometry nature simplest, most direct awakening invitation. Requires no technical knowledge, initiations, complex theories. Requires only eyes see, heart feel. Seeing geometry flower, see not just flower—see soul reflection. Recognizing leaf symmetry, recognize own internal order. Contemplating shell spiral, hear universe sound spinning within own being.

Arcturians affirm all true spiritual awakening begins this recognition: light is everything. Nature, silent beauty, saying this constantly. Geometry language uniting all things. Learning listen it, being not just understands world—remembers part it, one everything exists. Flower doesn't ask beautiful. Tree doesn't doubt place. Mountain doesn't fear falling. All follow geometry. Trust pattern. Pattern same living each human. Difference human can forget. Nature, never.

Hence, heals. Teaches. Mirror divine. Because in it, geometry isn't theory—living presence, wordless prayer, wall-less temple. Living this gaze, world transforms. Everything vibrates meaning. Shines order. Breathes together. Soul, finally, recognizes self part great creation design. Whole. Geometric. Sacred. Eternal.

Chapter 30
Conclusion and Continuity

Continuity sacred path defined not endpoint, living integration what experienced what still pulses come. Wisdom shared throughout journey, intertwined Arcturian codes, elevated frequency geometries, establishes active vibrational field, expanding beyond pages, symbols, words. Each reader traversing path leaves not entered; carries now new perception configuration, energy body restructured subtle revelations, silent practices operating levels beyond mind. Knowledge not just transmitted, activated—awakening ancient memories, recalibrating energy centers, strengthening bridge human, divine each being.

Experience lived here reveals continuous initiation, where sacred geometry assumes soul language role, cosmos hidden structure. Recognizing patterns, contemplating forms, allowing feel vibration, reader led expanded consciousness state. No doctrine need, belief imposition: knowing emerged within, nourished subtle contact broader consciousnesses serving catalysts, not authority. Path formed not disciples, reminded inherent mastery. Mastery now becomes basis next expansion cycle, cycle sacred lived naturally, each gesture, choice, silence imbued meaning, presence.

Journey conclusion, far from marking end, invites new way being world—more awake, coherent, luminous. Insights, activations echoing reading continue unfold, concentric waves touching ever deeper being layers. Integration happens not once, gradual flourishing, guided own inner wisdom. Each symbol remains portal revisitable; each practice, key usable again access refined connection states. In this state continuous presence true purpose reveals: be conscious light channel, live harmony universe rhythms, co-create realities aligned love frequency.

Geometry, revealed light, consciousness language, fulfilled key role here. Each chapter, door. Symbol, bridge. Practice, silent activation. Now, sacred path end, being invited not stop, but continue. Continue walking more presence, perceiving more clarity, being more truth. Because sacred isn't kept—lived. Lived, transforms everything.

Path purpose not just transmit knowledge. Not teach fixed truths, impose doctrines. What offered here reconnection. Reunion what already inhabited each being: heart knowing, Higher Self voice, spirit geometry. Arcturians placed not masters, mirrors. Mirrors reflecting light, allowed each see own essence forms previously dormant.

Sacred geometry, unveiled step-by-step book, showed not theory, living practice. Circle spiral, triangle cube, sound light, flower cosmos, each symbol reminder everything connected. No separation matter, spirit, heaven, earth, human, divine. Everything pulses unity, geometry that pulsing alphabet.

Arcturians transmitted codes, practices, symbols, visions not closed maps, seeds. Each reader now gardener own expansion. Each practice transform, symbol reveal new aspects, meditation infinitely deepened. Because true knowing doesn't end—unfolds, Flower Life petals, revealing new patterns being opens light.

Journey traversing healing, manifestation, ascension, Higher Self, Earth reconnection planes, brought forth deep call: call spiritual sovereignty. Arcturians came not create followers, awaken masters. Masters self. Beings walking vibrational autonomy, aligning Source freedom, building own inner temples, illuminating world simple coherent presence.

What spiritual sovereignty else live constant dialogue light? Not separate, part own being. Sovereign know self connected. No longer seek outside what vibrates inside. Honor each path step humility, firmness. Welcome other divine extension. Serve Earth gratitude. Love measureless, love highest geometry base frequency.

Light circles now forming planet wide—presential encounters, meditation groups, intuitive sharing, healing networks—reflection this vibrational continuity. Each elevating being, elevates field. Individual awakening impacts collective mesh. Arcturians remain present, not external guides, active consciousness subtle web enveloping Earth. Mission assist, sustain, inspire—never replace.

Book, then, doesn't end. Transforms practice. Incarnates daily life. Becomes silent prayer waking, sacred gesture touching water, gratitude eating, presence breathing, light gazing. Everything ritual. Sacred. Interlinked invisible patterns now perceived crystalline clarity.

Those wishing deepen, infinite paths. Codes redrawn, meditated, combined. Geometries explored new dimensions, meditations. Light language continues reveal who remains listening. Arcturian connection become more intimate, direct, vibrant. Just intention, surrender, love. Because contact frequency isn't technological—spiritual. Most powerful channel remains heart.

Continuity also manifests Earth cycles. Solstices, equinoxes, lunar phases, celestial events—all invitations renew connection, reactivate codes, realign field. Sacred spaces strengthened new practices. Daily rituals gain new meanings. Seeds planted book flourish new creations, circles, service manifestations.

Call now simple, profound: live geometric consciousness. See beauty forms. Feel order cycles. Honor light everything. Create intention. Love presence. Serve joy. Thus, continuity won't effort—flow. Dance. Expansion.

Arcturians conclude transmission reverence. Don't say goodbye. Say: "We are with you." Because don't depart. Remain vibration, light, fertile silence. Whenever heart opens, field aligns, intention pure, they'll be there—not above, outside, but beside. As siblings. Mirrors. Same Whole extension.

Closing book, something remains open: being own portal. Temple always there, waiting inhabited.

Light never extinguished, just awaited remembered. Geometry pulsing chest, awaiting lived. Because sacred is now. Path continues. And you are light it illuminates.

Epilogue

Some journeys lead us down unexpected paths. And there are those that silently guide us back to what we never stopped being. This reading was not just an intellectual journey—it was an energetic crossing. A dive into frequencies that lay dormant, awaiting the right moment for activation. And now that you have arrived here, something inside you is no longer the same.

It is impossible to pass through this field of wisdom without being deeply touched. The sacred geometry pulsating in each chapter was not limited to the pages. It restructured internal patterns, aligned forgotten rhythms, and returned to your consciousness an ancestral memory that words can never describe. You might still not understand everything rationally—and that's okay. Because what was activated, was activated in soul time.

What was revealed needs no external proof. The language of light echoing between the lines of this book spoke to your essence, not your paradigms. The symbols, sounds, portals described are not concepts—they are experiences. And more than that, they are mirrors. Mirrors of your stellar origin, your internal geometry, your capacity to manifest reality from vibration.

Now, perhaps more than ever, you understand that awakening is not a destination—it is a stance towards life. And that the Arcturians, with their subtle and loving presence, are not here to lead you, but to remind you that you always knew the way. They do not impose. They resonate. And by resonating, awaken. Like the bell echoing in an empty temple, suddenly revealing its vastness.

If you were touched, it's because you were ready. Ready to see beyond form. Ready to feel the invisible. Ready to listen to the silent song emanating from your being's center—which for millennia echoed among stars, waiting to be heard again here, on Earth, by you.

The transformation this book proposes is subtle, yet profound. It's not about abandoning the world, but inhabiting it with another consciousness. Understanding that matter isn't opposed to spirit—it's its densest expression. That each daily gesture, breath, silence, can be sacred geometry in motion. That you are, indeed, a living temple.

Light, now, is no longer just a distant idea. It is a state of presence. A technology pulsing in your field, ready to be used with every choice you make aligned with truth. You learned, here, that intention shapes reality. That sound reorganizes form. That the heart is the portal. And that ascension isn't escape—it's deep dive into totality of what one is.

This book ends, but what it awakened continues. Because true learning isn't pages—it's how you integrate them. How you breathe after reading. How you look sky, water, stones, people. How you perceive self part living, intelligent, harmonic network, dancing sphere symphony, vibrating creation patterns.

You now possess keys. Not open external doors, but remember you are portal itself. Everything revealed here—symbols, teachings, archetypes, cycles—soul tools. Maps, compasses, mirrors. At your disposal, not dogmas, invitations. And invitation clear: continue. Continue expanding. Listening. Trusting synchronicities, messages arriving dreams, geometries emerging daily life, subtle sensations touching heart without apparent reason. This language light action. New human born you.

Arcturians follow beside—not distant masters, frequencies resonating highest being part. Don't depart, because never arrived. Always here, waiting right moment you recognize not outside something, what vibrates purest interior.

Journey just beginning. Now, you have codes. Practices. Consciousness. Presence. Forgetting time dissolving. Remembrance time starts pulsing stronger. May you continue walking awakened heart. Existence geometry vibrate harmony stars. Voice sing spirit melody. Light inspire others also remember. And if one day, silence, feel again inexplicable call pulsing chest... know: journey continues. And you never alone.

www.ingramcontent.com/pod-product-compliance
Lightning Source LLC
LaVergne TN
LVHW090359210926
848480LV00002B/395